Periodontal Review

PERIODONTAL
REVIEW

Deborah A. Termeie, DDS

Clinical Lecturer
Department of Periodontics
School of Dentistry
University of California, Los Angeles
Los Angeles, California

Quintessence Publishing Co, Inc

Chicago, Berlin, Tokyo, London, Paris, Milan, Barcelona, Beijing, Istanbul, Moscow, New Delhi, Prague, São Paulo, Seoul, Singapore, and Warsaw

Library of Congress Cataloging-in-Publication Data

Termeie, Deborah.
  Periodontal review : a study guide / Deborah Termeie.
      p. ; cm.
  Includes bibliographical references and index.
  ISBN 978-0-86715-591-4 (softcover)
  I. Title.
  [DNLM: I. Periodontal Diseases--Examination Questions. 2. Periodontics--Examination Questions. 3. Periodontium--Examination Questions. WU 18.2]
    LC Classification not assigned
    617.6'320076--dc23
                                    2012051022

© 2013 Quintessence Publishing Co, Inc

Quintessence Publishing Co, Inc
4350 Chandler Drive
Hanover Park, IL 60133
www.quintpub.com

5 4 3 2

Editor: Bryn Grisham
Design: Ted Pereda
Production: Angelina Sanchez

Printed in the USA

Contents

Foreword

Becoming certified by the American Board of Periodontology (ABP) is an immense honor and an outward sign of a dedication to the specialty of periodontics and a drive to excel within the profession. According to the American Academy of Periodontology, the ABP "evaluates standards of periodontic practice by examining the qualifications and competence of periodontists who voluntarily apply to the board for certification as diplomates." After successful completion of a written qualifying examination, a candidate is considered *board eligible* and must then complete an oral examination in a defined period of time. The ABP defines a *diplomate* as "a periodontist who has made significant achievements beyond the mandatory educational requirements of the specialty and who is certified by the ABP." This reinforces board certification as a sign of dedication to the specialty and of committment to become the best periodontist possible.

To be educationally qualified for board certification, a candidate must be a certified dentist who has completed an accredited 3-year educational program in periodontology. The written and oral board examinations are comprehensive, covering all phases of periodontal health and disease and its diagnosis, treatment, and evaluation. In fact, the mission of the ABP is to "advance the art and science of periodontics and elevate the quality of periodontal care through the examination, certification, and recertification of periodontists and by encouraging the achievement and maintenance of diplomate status." Thus, one can appreciate that mastery of the body of knowledge required to complete the written and oral examinations is intimidating and overwhelming! *Periodontal Review* by Dr Deborah Termeie is an organized, detailed, and well-documented compilation of information designed to help candidates navigate the board certification examinations.

There are many periodontal specialty programs across the United States, and while each covers the components mandated by the Commission on Dental Accreditation of the American Dental Association, variation exists between programs because of different faculties and diverse patient experiences. Therefore, a comprehensive well-documented study guide can help standardize the information provided in the various educational programs. More important, the body of knowledge that one must know to become board certified is overwhelming, and as more publications in the peer-reviewed literature become available every year, this body of knowledge grows exponentially. Learning the necessary material seems impossible. These are just two reasons why this study guide is helpful.

In the past, study to become board certified would require months of preparation just to figure out how to organize the literature to understand the critical information. Dr Termeie has done this task for you. Chapters cover diverse topics of periodontolgy, including health and disease conditions and therapeutic options, and the information is presented in an easy-to-understand question and answer format. The detail for treatment options alone is impressive; it includes nonsurgical and surgical therapy, chemotherapeutics, lasers, occlusal therapy, and bone and implant therapy for replacing missing teeth. Dr Termeie includes other material relevant to the board candidate, such as evidence-based medicine and dentistry, related human physiology and pathology, pharmacology, and oral medicine and pathology.

Another helpful aspect to this study guide is that Dr Termeie often provides data for and against a question in a concise and understandable format. Additionally, simple diagrams, tables, and charts are used throughout, which makes the text easy to understand even when discussing difficult topics. Dr Termeie also provides clinical examples that demonstrate how patient cases are documented and presented during the board examinations.

Collectively this study guide provides a comprehensive and well-organized review of major concepts in the field of periodontology and can be used either to start the studying process or as a self-examination review prior to taking the examinations. I believe that this study guide will be an essential tool for anyone who is going through the periodontal certifying board examinations or the board recertification examination or who would like to have a comprehensive reference guide in periodontology. I would like to thank Dr Termeie for the time and effort that she expended to compile this information and for making it comprehensive, organized, and easy to understand. Present and future periodontal diplomates will be much better prepared due to this effort by Dr Termeie.

David L. Cochran, DDS, MS, PhD, MMSci
Proud Diplomate of the American Board of Periodontology

Professor and Chairman
Department of Periodontics
Dental School
The University of Texas Health Science Center at San Antonio
San Antonio, Texas

Preface

As periodontal residency graduates embark on their journey to board certification, many of them come face to face with a plethora of study materials and information but no comprehensive study resource designed to help them prepare for their examinations. *Periodontal Review* was specifically written to address this void.

The material in this book is presented in a question and answer format for ease of study. The classic literature is cited as well as more recent and practical literature on topics such as diagnosis, nonsurgical therapy, surgical therapy, regeneration, and implants. Literature evidence for opposing viewpoints is also presented throughout the book. Additionally, each chapter contains clear and relevant tables, illustrations, and pictures. This comprehensive and yet concise approach to periodontics is aimed at preparing the candidate for periodontal examinations and clinical practice.

Periodontal Review is a useful resource for residents, practicing periodontists preparing for board certification, dental students, and dental hygiene students seeking a broader appreciation and in-depth understanding of periodontics. Topics chosen are those emphasized in periodontal residency graduation examinations as well as the oral examination of the American Board of Periodontology.

Acknowledgments

I would like to acknowledge my mentors—Philip R. Melnick, DDS; Thomas N. Sims, DDS; Paulo M. Camargo, DDS; and Thomas Han, DDS—for their guidance and advice. I would also like to thank my program director at UCLA, Perry R. Klokkevold, DDS. Lastly, I would like to thank my loving husband, David, and my children, Gabriella and Elliot. Without their love and support, this book would not have been possible.

About the Author

Deborah A. Termeie, DDS, is a clinical instructor in the Department of Periodontics at UCLA in Los Angeles, California. She is a diplomate of the American Board of Periodontology (ABP), and it was her experience preparing for the ABP qualifying exams that inspired her to write this book. Dr Termeie has published on the topic of evidence-based dentistry and is the recipient of several awards, including the Excellence in Implantology Research award from the California Society of Periodontics. She maintains a private practice in Beverly Hills, California.

Evidence-Based Dentistry

Background

Q: What is the evidence-based approach?

Evidence-based dentistry is the merging of clinically pertinent scientific evidence to the patient's oral and medical condition and history. The dentist uses the evidence to make sound decisions about diagnosis, prognosis, and treatment.

Q: What is the PICO question?

The *PICO question* is a question that includes a *population* to be examined, the nature of the *intervention* to be inspected, a *comparison* statement, and the type of *outcome* to be evaluated. It should be problem-focused and concise.

Example: In patients with periodontitis (population), what is the effect of osseous surgery (intervention) compared with controls (comparison) on clinical and patient-centered outcomes (outcome)?

Q: What is the step-by-step process for making an evidence-based decision in a dental practice?

The steps involved in evidence-based decision making in a dental practice are shown in Fig 1-1.

| Formulate a PICO question | Research the PICO question and collect evidence | Analyze the data that has been collected | Apply the data to the dental practice | Evaluate the results |

Fig 1-1 Evidence-based decision making. (Based on data in Chiappelli et al.[1])

Studies

Q: What are the different study types (ranked from highest level of evidence to lowest)?

The different types of studies are shown, ranked in order of highest to lowest level of evidence, in Fig 1-2.

Systematic reviews and meta-analyses

Randomized and controlled clinical trials
(Patients are randomly placed in test or control groups)

Controlled trials not randomized

Cohort studies
(Analytic studies in which patients are studied longitudinally)

Case-control studies
(Observational studies that have test and control groups; usually retrospective)

Cross-sectional studies
(Studies done at one time point)

Case report studies

Fig 1-2 Different studies ranked from highest level of evidence to lowest. (Based on Chiappelli et al.[2])

Q: **Describe the difference between a cross-sectional study and a longitudinal study.**

A cross-sectional study is done at one time point, whereas a longitudinal study ranges over a period of time, allowing temporal relationships to be investigated.

Q: **What is the *P* value?**

The *P* value is the probability of obtaining a test statistic at least as extreme as the one observed, assuming that the null hypothesis is true. The smaller the *P* value, the less likely the effect was due to chance.

Q: **What is the difference between internal and external validity?**

The difference between internal and external validity is shown in Fig 1-3.

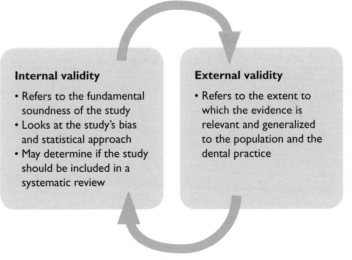

Internal validity

- Refers to the fundamental soundness of the study
- Looks at the study's bias and statistical approach
- May determine if the study should be included in a systematic review

External validity

- Refers to the extent to which the evidence is relevant and generalized to the population and the dental practice

Fig 1-3 Internal and external validity.

References

1. Chiappelli F, Brant XMC, Oluwadara OO, Neagos N, Ramchandani MH. Introduction: Research synthesis in evidence-based clinical decision-making. In: Chiappelli F, Brant XMC, Neagos N, Oluwadara OO, Ramchandani MH (eds). Evidence-Based Practice: Toward Optimizing Clinical Outcomes. London: Springer, 2010:5.
2. Nocini PF, Verlato G, De Santis D, et al. Strengths and limitations of the evidence-based movement aimed to improve clinical outcomes in dentistry and oral surgery. In: Chiappelli F, Brant XMC, Neagos N, Oluwadara OO, Ramchandani MH (eds). Evidence-Based Practice: Toward Optimizing Clinical Outcomes. London: Springer, 2010:151.

2

Periodontal Anatomy

Anatomy

Q: Identify the anatomical structures of the periodontium shown below.

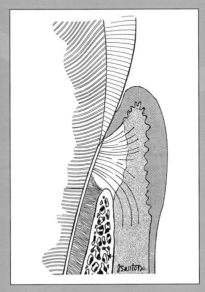

Fig 2-1a Illustration of the periodontium. (Reprinted from Fan and Berry[1] with permission.)

The answers are shown on the next page in Fig 2-1b.

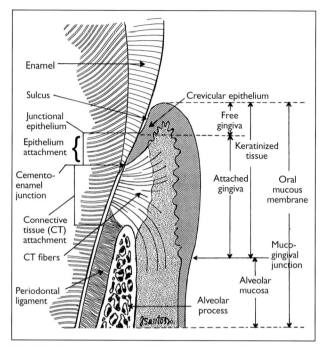

Fig 2-1b Labeled anatomy of the periodontium. (Reprinted from Fan and Berry[1] with permission.)

Q: Where does the vascular supply of the periodontium originate?

The external carotid artery and its main branches, which include the lingual, facial, and maxillary arteries, are the vascular supply for the periodontium. Locally, the blood supply comes from the supraperiosteal vessels and vessels from the periodontal ligament (PDL) and bone.[2]

Q: What is the main innervation for the periodontium?

The trigeminal nerve and its branches provide the main innervation for the periodontium.

Definitions

Q: What is attached gingiva?

The *attached gingiva* is the area from the base of the sulcus to the mucogingival junction. It prevents the free gingiva from being separated from the tooth. Its height is determined by subtracting the sulcus probing depth from the total width of the keratinized tissue. It consists of thick lamina propria and deep rete pegs. Goaslind et al[3] reported that the attached gingival thickness is 1.25 ± 0.42 mm.

Q: What is keratinized attached gingiva?

The *keratinized attached gingiva* is that found from the gingival margin to the mucogingival junction.

Q: Define alveolar mucosa.

Alveolar mucosa is the covering of the alveolar process that is nonkeratinized, unstippled, and movable. It extends from the mucogingival junction to the floor of the mouth and vestibular epithelium.

Q: What is clinical attachment loss (CAL)?

If the marginal gingiva is below the cementoenamel junction (CEJ):

CAL = pocket depth + [CEJ to marginal gingiva]

If the marginal gingiva is above the CEJ:

CAL = [marginal gingiva to CEJ] – [marginal gingiva to bottom of pocket]

Q: What is Ante's law?

Ante's law states that the root surface area of the abutment teeth must be equal to or greater than that of teeth being replaced with pontics. This helps determine the number of abutments needed for a fixed partial denture.

Gingival Epithelium

Q: What are the characteristics of healthy gingiva?

Healthy gingiva is coral pink, firm, follows the CEJ of the teeth, and may be stippled. The color of the gingiva is associated with the pigmentation of the patient. In dark-haired individuals, the gingiva can be darker than that in blond patients.

Q: What are the five types of gingival fibers?

There are five types of gingival fibers:

1. Dentogingival group: There are three types of fibers within this group.
   - Fibers extending coronally toward the gingival crest
   - Fibers extending laterally to the facial gingival surface
   - Fibers extending horizontally beyond the alveolar crest height and then apically along the alveolar bone cortex
2. Alveologingival group: Fibers in this group run coronally into the lamina propria from the periosteum at the alveolar crest.
3. Dentoperiosteal fibers: These fibers insert into the periosteum of the alveolar crest and fan out to the adjacent cementum.
4. Circular group: These are the only fibers that are confined to the gingiva and do not attach to the teeth.
5. Transseptal group: These fibers bridge the interproximal tissue between adjacent teeth and insert into the cementum.

Q: What is the composition of the oral mucosa (the tissue lining the oral cavity)?

The oral mucosa is composed of masticatory, lining, and specialized tissues (Fig 2-2).

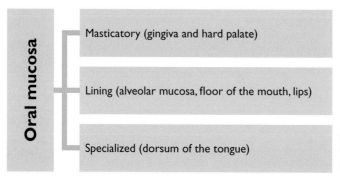

Oral mucosa
- Masticatory (gingiva and hard palate)
- Lining (alveolar mucosa, floor of the mouth, lips)
- Specialized (dorsum of the tongue)

Fig 2-2 Composition of the oral mucosa. (Based on Avery.[4])

Q: What is the composition of the gingival epithelium?

The gingival epithelium consists of oral (masticatory), oral sulcular, and junctional epithelia (Fig 2-3).

Oral (masticatory) epithelium	Oral sulcular epithelium	Junctional epithelum
• Orthokeratinized, stratified squamous • Surface cells lose their nuclei and contain keratin • Made of the following: free gingiva (base of the sulcus to the free gingival margin, ie, the most coronal part of the gingiva), attached gingiva, and palatal tissue	• Epithelium that lines the sulcus • No rete pegs in healthy tissue	• Attaches to the tooth via a hemidesmosomal layer and a basal lamina • Nonkeratinized and has a fast turnover • Permeable • Most apical part lies at the CEJ in healthy tissue

Fig 2-3 Composition of the gingival epithelium. (Based on Clerehugh et al.[5])

Q: Describe the four layers of cells that comprise the masticatory epithelium.

There are four layers of cells that comprise the masticatory epithelium[2]:

1. Stratum basale: Cuboidal cells found at the basement membrane; epithelial cell replication takes place in this location. This layer contains melanocytes and Merkel cells.
2. Stratum spinosum: The "spines" are desmosomes allowing intracellular contacts. It is the thickest layer and contains Langerhans cells, which are derived from bone marrow and take part in immune surveillance.
3. Stratum granulosum: Cells in this layer appear flat. Keratinocytes migrating from the underlying stratum spinosum become known as *granular cells* in this layer. These cells contain keratohyalin granules, protein structures that promote hydration and cross-linking of keratin.
4. Stratum corneum: Outermost layer containing dead cells and consisting of ortho- and parakeratinization. It is composed of compactly packed tonofilaments.

Q: Where are the widest and narrowest zones of gingiva?

The average thickness of the gingiva is 1.25 mm.[3] The widest zone of gingiva is in the maxillary anterior region; the narrowest zone is at the facial aspect of the mandibular first premolar.[2]

Connective Tissue

Q: What is the composition of connective tissue?

Connective tissue is fibrous, consisting of mostly type I collagen, ground substances, and mucopolysaccharides. It also contains white blood cells, blood vessels, lymphatics, and nerves.[2]

Q: What determines whether epithelium is keratinized or nonkeratinized?

The underlying connective tissue determines whether the epithelium is keratinized.[6]

Periodontal Ligament (PDL)

Q: Where is the average width of the PDL greatest and where is it narrowest?

The width of the PDL is greatest at the apex and narrowest in the middle. Older individuals have thicker fiber bundles in the PDL than younger individuals. The average width of the PDL is 0.2 mm.

Q: What provides the blood supply to the PDL?

Superior and inferior alveolar arteries provide the blood supply to the PDL, which is a vascular tissue.

Q: What are the functions of the PDL?

• Protect vessels and nerves
• Transmit occlusal forces
• Attach the tooth to bone
• Perform formative and remodeling functions

Q: What are the fibers of the PDL?

The fibers of the PDL include the alveolar crest, horizontal, oblique (most numerous), interradicular, and apical fibers.

Q: Describe and define ankylosis.

Ankylosis is the fusion of the cementum and alveolar bone with obliteration of the PDL. It develops after chronic periapical inflammation, tooth reimplantation, and occlusal trauma.

Alveolar Bone

Q: What is the composition of alveolar bone?

Alveolar bone consists of[2]:

- Cortical bone
- Cancellous trabeculae (more prevalent in the maxilla)
- Alveolar bone proper (lines the tooth socket)

Q: What are the functions of the alveolar bone?

The alveolar bone has three functions[2]:

1. Protection
2. Support
3. Calcium metabolism

Cementum

Q: Where are acellular cementum and cellular cementum located?

Acellular cementum is located on the enamel at the CEJ. It does not contain cementocytes and forms slowly.

Cellular cementum is located at the apical third of the root. It is more irregular and forms rapidly. With age, there is an increase in width of the cellular cementum.

Q: **What percentage of the cementum and enamel overlap?**

- 60% of the cementum and enamel overlap.
- 30% of the cementum and enamel form a butt joint.
- 10% of the cementum and enamel are separated by a gap.

Q: **What is the difference between extrinsic and intrinsic cementum?**

Extrinsic fibers are made of Sharpey fibers from the PDL, whereas intrinsic fibers are cementum fibers produced by cementoblasts (Fig 2-4).

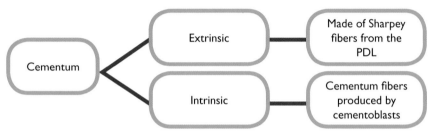

Fig 2-4 Characteristics of extrinsic and intrinsic cementum.

Q: **How does the junctional epithelium attach to the cementum?**

The junctional epithelium attaches to the cementum via hemidesmosomes and replicates every 5 days.

Temporomandibular Joint (TMJ)

Q: **What is the composition of the TMJ disc (meniscus)?**

The TMJ disc is composed of dense connective tissue.

Q: **Describe the movement of the TMJ.**

The meniscus divides the joint into two compartments. The upper compartment has translational movement, and the lower compartment has rotational movement.

Q: What is meniscal derangement with and without reduction?

- With reduction: The disc as well as the posterior band of the meniscus is anteriorly displaced in front of the condyle upon opening. This causes a popping or clicking sound.
- Without reduction: In some patients, the meniscus remains anteriorly displaced at full opening. This is a much more serious condition.

Collagen

Q: Describe the four different types of collagen.

- Type I. Skin, tendon, vascular ligature, organs, bone (main component of the organic part of bone)
- Type II: Cartilage (main component of cartilage)
- Type III: Comprised of reticular fibers, commonly found alongside type I collagen, found mostly in smooth muscle
- Type IV: Forms basis of cell basement membrane

Biologic Width

Q: What is biologic width?

The *biologic width* is defined as the physiologic dimension of the junctional epithelium and connective tissue attachment. It is measured from the most coronal part of the junctional epithelium to the crest of the alveolar bone. In studies on cadavers, Gargiulo[7] found a connective tissue attachment of 1.07 mm and a junctional epithelium attachment of 0.97 mm. Therefore, the biologic width is about 2 mm. He also found the sulcus, which is not part of the biologic width, to be 0.69 mm.

Q: What results from violation of the biologic width?

If subgingival restorations violate the biologic width, periodontal bone loss and inflammation may occur. The body will try to make room between the margin of the restoration and the alveolar bone to allow for reestablishment of the biologic width.

Miscellaneous

Q: What is the most common area of recurrent pockets?

The mesial aspect of the maxillary first premolars and first molars are the most common areas of recurrent pockets.

Q: Which muscles elevate and depress the mandible?

- Elevate: Temporalis, medial pterygoid, and masseter
- Depress: Lateral pterygoid, digastric, and mylohyoid

References

1. Fan PP, Berry TG. Cast-gold restorations. In: Summitt JB, Robbins JW, Hilton TJ, Schwartz RS (eds). Fundamentals of Operative Dentistry: A Contemporary Approach, ed 3. Chicago: Quintessence, 2006:543.
2. Serio FG, Hawley C. Manual of Clinical Periodontics. Hudson, OH: Lexi-Comp, 2002.
3. Goaslind GD, Robertson PB, Mahan CJ, Morrison WW, Olson JV. Thickness of facial gingiva. J Periodontol 1977;48:768–771.
4. Avery J. Oral Development and Histology, ed 3. Stuttgart, Germany: Thieme Medical, 2002:250.
5. Clerehugh V, Tugnait A, Genco RJ. Periodontology at a Glance. Oxford: Wiley-Blackwell, 2009:3.
6. Karring T, Lang NP, Löe H. The role of gingival connective tissue in determining epithelial differentiation. J Periodontal Res 1975;10:1–11.
7. Gargiulo AW. Dimensions and relations of the dentogingival junction in humans. J Periodontol 1961;32:261–267.

3

Furcations

Background

Q: What is the prevalence of furcation involvement?

In a study on periodontal patients, Svärdström and Wennström[1] found a greater prevalence of furcation involvement in maxillary molars than in mandibular molars. The narrowest furcation entrance was found on the buccal aspect of maxillary and mandibular molars, and the highest frequency of involvement was the distal aspect of the maxillary first molar. The mesial aspect of the second molar had the least frequency of furcation involvement.

Q: What is a furcation fornix?

The *furcation fornix* is the roof of the furcation.

Q: Is the Nabers probe a valid and efficient tool for detecting furcation invasion?

Eickholz and Kim[2] found that the Nabers Probe, marked in 3-mm increments, is a valid method of diagnosing furcation lesions.

Classification

Q: Describe the Hamp classification.

The classification by Hamp et al[3] involves a horizontal measurement:

- F0: No furcation involvement.
- F1: The probe can penetrate the furcation less than 3 mm.
- F2: The furcation can be probed greater than 3 mm, but it is not a through and through furcation involvement.
- F3: Through and through furcation involvement.

Q: Describe the Glickman classification.

The Glickman[4] classification is presented in Fig 3-1.

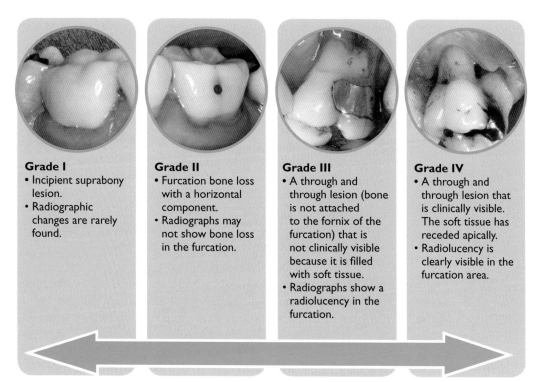

Grade I
- Incipient suprabony lesion.
- Radiographic changes are rarely found.

Grade II
- Furcation bone loss with a horizontal component.
- Radiographs may not show bone loss in the furcation.

Grade III
- A through and through lesion (bone is not attached to the fornix of the furcation) that is not clinically visible because it is filled with soft tissue.
- Radiographs show a radiolucency in the furcation.

Grade IV
- A through and through lesion that is clinically visible. The soft tissue has receded apically.
- Radiolucency is clearly visible in the furcation area.

Fig 3-1 Glickman classification.

Q: Describe the Tarnow classification.

The classification by Tarnow and Fletcher[5] is a subclassification of the Glickman furcation classification that measures the vertical probing depth from the roof of the furca:

- A: 0 to 3 mm
- B: 4 to 6 mm
- C: Greater than 7 mm

Treatment Options

Q: What are the treatment options for furcation defects?

- Nonsurgical debridement
- Surgical debridement
- Surgical exposure of the furcation
- Regeneration (guided tissue regeneration [GTR] and enamel matrix derivative [EMD])
- Extraction
- Root resection
- Tunnel preparation

Q: Is open/closed flap scaling and root planing effective in furcation lesions?

A review by Cobb[6] demonstrated a less favorable response to scaling and root planing by molars with furcation involvement compared with those without furcation lesions and single-rooted teeth. He surmised that this was related to the inability to remove all pathogenic microbial flora due to the furcal anatomy restricting access for mechanical therapy.

Bower[7] found that 81% of the time the furcation entrance is 1 mm or less. The study also found that 58% of the time the furcation entrance is 0.7 mm or less. The blade width of commonly used periodontal curettes is 0.75 mm. The ultrasonic (smaller) tip would fit better than the tip of a Gracey curette in a grade II or III furcation.

Wylam et al[8] found no significant difference between open and closed flap root planing. The study further concluded that root planing is inefficient in the debridement of furcation lesions and does not allow for periodontal regeneration.

Q: Can a grade II furcation be treated successfully? Which treatment is the most effective?

Evans et al[9] reviewed 50 papers that studied 1,016 grade II furcations. The teeth had received various treatments such as bone grafts, open flap debridement, and GTR. The study found complete closure of the furcation in 20% of the grade II furcations and an improvement of a grade II to a grade I furcation in 33% of the cases. In general, there was a 50% improvement for grade II furcations. The most effective treatment was a bone graft with GTR, and the least effective treatment was open flap debridement (2% of the grade II furcations had complete closure).

Bowers et al[10] discovered complete closure of grade II mandibular furcations in 50% of patients. There was a 68% improvement of a grade II to a grade I furcation.

Murphy and Gunsolley[11] performed a systematic review and discovered that GTR is more effective than open flap debridement in the treatment of furcation defects. The study also found that in furcation lesions vertical probing depth, vertical probing attachment levels, and horizontal open probing attachment levels—but no intrabony outcomes—were improved by augmentation with a particulate graft in conjunction with the GTR barrier.

Q: What factors influence the success of treatment?

Bowers et al[10] found poorer results in the treatment of furcation lesions in smokers. Smokers had a 62.5% chance of having a class II residual defect compared with nonsmokers, who had a 14.3% chance. Furcation fill decreases at an increased horizontal and vertical presurgical probing attachment level (greater than 5 mm). The following were found to reduce the frequency of clinical closure:

- Increased distance between the roof of the furcation and the crest of bone
- Increased distance between the roof of the furcation and the base of the defect
- The depth of the horizontal defect
- Increased divergence of roots at the crest of bone

Q: Are teeth that undergo the tunnel preparation in the furcation area prone to caries?

Hellden et al[12] studied 156 teeth with advanced periodontal furcation defects that were treated by tunnel preparations. The study found that 25% of the teeth developed caries.

A retrospective study by Feres et al[13] demonstrated that a history of root caries was the only factor with a positive association with caries incidence in tunnels.

Q: Are biologic mediators effective in furcation lesions?

- EMD: A study by Araújo and Lindhe[14] used EMD and a barrier in the test defects and just a barrier in control defects. The test defect was found to have acellular cementum in the apical portion, while in the coronal portion a thick cellular cementum, similar to the cementum found in the control group, was detected. Both the test and control group furcation defects were found to be clinically closed and to contain bone and periodontal ligament tissue that appeared structurally similar to newly formed root cementum.
- Recombinant human osteogenic protein-1 (OP-1): Giannobile et al[15] found distinct stimulation of osteogenesis, regenerative cementum, and new attachment formation in sites treated with three different concentrations of OP-1.
- Platelet-rich plasma (PRP): Pradeep et al[16] reported that although the degree II status of the studied furcation defects was unchanged, sites treated with PRP showed a statistically significant difference in all clinical and radiographic parameters compared with those receiving open flap debridement.

Anatomical Factors

Q: What anatomical factors are associated with furcation lesions?

The anatomical factors associated with furcation lesions are shown in Fig 3-2.

Fig 3-2 Anatomical factors associated with furcation lesions.

Q: What percentage of molars have accessory canals in the furcation?

Gutmann[17] studied 102 molars and found that 28.4% (29.4% of mandibular molars and 27.4% of maxillary molars) have accessory canals in the furcation.

Q: What is the classification for cervical enamel projections?

Masters and Hoskins[18] classified cervical enamel projections as follows:

- Grade 1: Extends from the CEJ to the furcation
- Grade 2: Approaches the furcation
- Grade 3: Extends into the furcation horizontally

Q: What is the frequency of cervical enamel projections?

Swan and Hurt[19] discovered that mandibular second molars had the highest incidence of cervical enamel projections (51.0%), while the lowest incidence was found in the maxillary first molars (13.6%). The most frequently encountered enamel projections in the study were grade 1, and the buccal surfaces were the most common location of cervical enamel projections.

Roussa[20] observed 60 teeth and discovered cervical enamel projections in 30% of the teeth examined.

Q: Is there a relationship between cervical enamel projections and furcations?

It is believed that the existence of cervical enamel projections inhibits connective tissue attachment and makes management of the furcation difficult.

Swan and Hurt[19] showed a positive correlation between grade 2 and grade 3 cervical enamel projections and periodontally involved furcations. However, the study did not find a relationship between grade 1 projections and furcation involvements.

A review by Lima and Hebling[21] found an association between cervical enamel projection, inflammatory periodontal disease, and molar furcation involvement.

Q: Describe how root concavities can affect prognosis of a tooth. Where are the concavities located on the first molars?

It is much more difficult to perform scaling and root planing on teeth with concavities, and as a result they can have a deleterious effect on the prognosis of a tooth. It is also challenging for the patient to maintain oral hygiene.

The root concavities for the first molars, as described by Bower,[22] are presented in Fig 3-3.

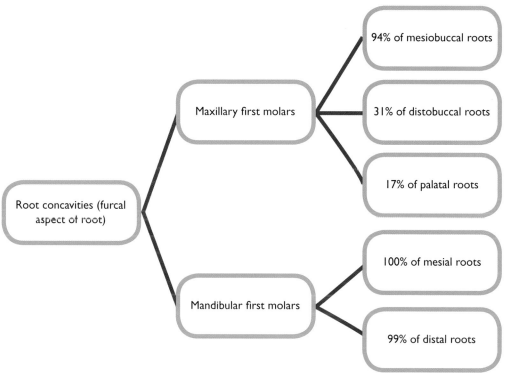

Fig 3-3 Anatomy of root concavities.

Q: **How do different furcations compare in regard to entrance width?**

The differences in furcation entrance width are as follows[22]:

• Mandibular molars: Buccal furcation entrance width is greater than lingual furcation entrance width.
• Maxillary molars: Mesial entrance width is greater than distal entrance width, which is greater than buccal entrance width.

Q: **Where are enamel pearls found most often? How can they contribute to furcation lesions?**

According to Moskow and Canut,[23] enamel pearls have a tendency to originate in the furcation areas of molars, especially the maxillary second and third molars. The study found an incidence of 1.1% to 9.7%.

As with cervical enamel projections, the existence of enamel pearls inhibits connective tissue attachment and makes management of the furcation difficult.

Q: How much attachment loss occurs for a furcation entrance to be observed in a maxillary molar?

According to Gher and Dunlap,[24] the mean distances from the CEJ to the mesial, facial, and distal furcation entrances are 3.6, 4.2, and 4.8 mm, respectively. Attachment loss of 6 mm is associated with a class III furcation.

Q: How much surface area does each of the maxillary roots comprise?

According to Hermann et al,[25] the roots comprise the following surface areas:

- Mesiobuccal: 36%
- Palatal: 35%
- Distobuccal: 28%

Q: What is an intermediate bifurcation ridge? How can it contribute to a furcation lesion?

Everett et al[26] first described the ridges. He studied 328 mandibular teeth and found that 73% had an intermediate bifurcation ridge, which is cementum extending from the mesial to the distal of a furcation opening on a mandibular molar. Its existence can hamper effective plaque control by the patient and the dentist.

Q: Describe cementicles and their contribution to furcation lesions.

Cementicles are calcified masses adherent to or separated from the tooth's root. Similar to intermediate bifurcation ridges, they compromise effective scaling and root planing by the dentist and oral hygiene by the patient.

Restorations

Q: Do restored molars have a higher percentage of furcation lesions than teeth without restorations?

Wang et al[27] demonstrated a higher percentage of furcation involvement but no greater mobility in molars with a crown or proximal restoration when compared with nonrestored molars. Restored molars also showed a greater mean probing periodontal attachment loss than nonrestored molars, but the difference was only marginally significant.

References

1. Svärdström G, Wennström JL. Prevalence of furcation involvements in patients referred for periodontal treatment. J Clin Periodontol 1996;23:1093–1099.
2. Eickholz P, Kim TS. Reproducibility and validity of the assessment of clinical furcation parameters as related to different probes. J Periodontol 1998;69:328–336.
3. Hamp SE, Nyman S, Lindhe J. Periodontal treatment of multirooted teeth. Results after 5 years. J Clin Periodontol 1975;2:126–135.
4. Glickman I. Clinical Periodontology: The Periodontium in Health and Disease; Recognition, Diagnosis and Treatment of Periodontal Disease in the Practice of General Dentistry. Philadelphia: Saunders, 1953.
5. Tarnow D, Fletcher P. Classification of the vertical component of furcation involvement. J Periodontol 1984;55:283–284.
6. Cobb CM. Non-surgical pocket therapy: Mechanical. Ann Periodontol 1996;1:443–490.
7. Bower RC. Furcation morphology relative to periodontal treatment. Furcation entrance architecture. J Periodontol 1979;50.23–27.
8. Wylam JM, Mealey BL, Mills MP, Waldrop TC, Moskowicz DC. The clinical effectiveness of open versus closed scaling and root planing on multi-rooted teeth. J Periodontol 1993;64:1023–1028.
9. Evans GH, Yukna RA, Gardiner DL, Cambre KM. Frequency of furcation closure with regenerative periodontal therapy. J West Soc Periodontol Periodontal Abstr 1996;44(4):101–109.
10. Bowers GM, Schallhorn RG, McClain PK, Morrison GM, Morgan R, Reynolds MA. Factors influencing the outcome of regenerative therapy in mandibular Class II furcations: Part I. J Periodontol 2003;74:1255–1268.
11. Murphy KG, Gunsolley JC. Guided tissue regeneration for the treatment of periodontal intrabony and furcation defects. A systematic review. Ann Periodontol 2003;8:266–302.
12. Hellden LB, Elliot A, Steffensen B, Steffensen JE. The prognosis of tunnel preparations in treatment of class III furcations. A follow-up study. J Periodontol 1989;60:182–187.
13. Feres M, Araujo MW, Figueiredo LC, Oppermann RV. Clinical evaluation of tunneled molars: A retrospective study. J Int Acad Periodontol 2006;8(3):96–103.
14. Araújo MG, Lindhe J. GTR treatment of degree III furcation defects following application of enamel matrix proteins. An experimental study in dogs. J Clin Periodontol 1998;25:524–530.
15. Giannobile WV, Ryan S, Shih MS, Su DL, Kaplan PL, Chan TC. Recombinant human osteogenic protein-1 (OP-1) stimulates periodontal wound healing in class III furcation defects. J Periodontol 1998;69:129–137.
16. Pradeep AR, Pai S, Garg G, Devi P, Shetty SK. A randomized clinical trial of autologous platelet-rich plasma in the treatment of mandibular degree II furcation defects. J Clin Periodontol 2009;36:581–588.
17. Gutmann JL. Prevalence, location, and patency of accessory canals in the furcation region of permanent molars. J Periodontol 1978;49:21–26.
18. Masters DH, Hoskins SW. Projection of cervical enamel into molar furcations. J Periodontol 1964;35:49–53.
19. Swan RH, Hurt WC. Cervical enamel projections as an etiologic factor in furcation involvement. J Am Dent Assoc 1976;93:342–345.
20. Roussa E. Anatomic characteristics of the furcation and root surfaces of molar teeth and their significance in the clinical management of marginal periodontitis. Clin Anat 1998;11:177–186.
21. Lima AF, Hebling E. Cervical enamel projection related to furcation involvement. Braz Dent J 1994;5:121–127.
22. Bower RC. Furcation morphology relative to periodontal treatment. Furcation root surface anatomy. J Periodontol 1979;50:366–374.
23. Moskow BS, Canut PM. Studies on root enamel (2). Enamel pearls. A review of their morphology, localization, nomenclature, occurrence, classification, histogenesis and incidence. J Clin Periodontol 1990;17:275–281.
24. Gher MW Jr, Dunlap RW. Linear variation of the root surface area of the maxillary first molar. J Periodontol 1985;56:39–43.
25. Hermann DW, Gher ME Jr, Dunlap RM, Pelleu GB Jr. The potential attachment area of the maxillary first molar. J Periodontol 1983;54:431–434.

26. Everett FG, Jump EB, Holder TD, Williams GC. The intermediate bifurcational ridge: A study of the morphology of the bifurcation of the lower first molar. J Dent Res 1958;37:162–169.
27. Wang HL, Burgett FG, Shyr Y. The relationship between restoration and furcation involvement on molar teeth. J Periodontol 1993;64:302–305.

Epidemiology and Etiology

Risk Factors and Risk Indicators

Q: What is the difference between a risk factor and a risk indicator?

A *risk factor* is a characteristic that places an individual at increased risk of contracting a disease. A *risk indicator* is a probable or putative risk factor that has been identified in cross-sectional correlation studies but not confirmed through longitudinal studies.

Q: What are the risk factors for periodontitis?

The risk factors for periodontitis are:

Tobacco use
- Strongest modifiable risk factor and predictor of future disease.
- According to Grossi,[1] smokers are 2.7 times more likely to have periodontal disease than nonsmokers.
- Smokers have 18 times more periodontal pathogens compared with nonsmokers.

Poor oral hygiene
- Listgarten[2] suggested increased plaque mass or reduced host defense may precipitate episodes of periodontal destruction.
- Löe et al[3] observed 480 tea plantation workers that were not exposed to preventive care for 15 years. They found that 8% of the population had rapid progression to periodontal disease, 11% had no progression, and 81% had moderate progression.

Diabetes
- Three times more bone loss and attachment loss has been found in patients with diabetes.
- After treatment of periodontal disease, there is a 10% drop in sugar levels.[4]

Genetics
- In a study by Kornman et al,[5] 86.0% of the severe periodontitis patients were either smokers or had the interleukin 1 genotype.
- According to Michalowicz et al,[6] 50% of enhanced risk for periodontitis can be accounted for by genetics alone.

Q: What are the risk indicators for periodontitis?

Following are the risk indicators for periodontitis:

- Age: Increased age is associated with increased extent and severity of chronic periodontitis.
- Sex: Male patients have poorer hygiene than female patients.
- Socioeconomic status: Those with lower socioeconomic status have less education and limited access to care.
- Race: There is a greater incidence of periodontitis in black and Hispanic populations. Blacks were found to be at much greater risk of aggressive periodontitis than whites.[7]
- Obesity: Adipose tissue can produce cytokines, which can lead to a hyperinflamed state. Gorman et al[8] found that overall obesity and central adiposity are associated with an increased hazard of periodontal disease progression in men.
- Alcohol: Shepherd[9] found evidence suggesting that alcohol consumption is a risk indicator for periodontitis. Longitudinal studies on the association of alcohol dependence and consumption with periodontitis are needed to confirm the association.
- Stress: Genco et al[10] found that financial stress and the coping mechanism of the patient were related to periodontal disease. They found that the effects of stress on periodontal disease can be moderated by adequate coping behaviors.

- Contraceptives: There is a possible association between injectable progesterone contraceptives and poor periodontal health, as indicated by a study
that found an increased likelihood of indicators of poor periodontal health,
including gingivitis and periodontitis, in women who had taken or were
currently taking depot medroxyprogesterone acetate (DMPA) injectable
contraceptives.[11]

Epidemiology Terminology

Q: What is an odds ratio?

An *odds ratio* is the probability that a person with an adverse outcome was
exposed to risk. An odds ratio that is greater than 1 has a positive association.

Q: What is the difference between sensitivity and specificity?

Sensitivity is the proportion of subjects with a disease who test positive, and
specificity is the proportion of subjects without the disease who test negative.

Q: What is the difference between prevalence and incidence?

Prevalence is defined as the total number of cases (or cases of the risk factor)
in the population at a given time, divided by the number of individuals in the
population. *Incidence* is a measure of the risk of developing a new condition
within a specified period of time.

Indices

Q: What is the Gingival Index?

The Gingival Index (Löe[12]) incorporates bleeding on probing and color
change:

- 0: Normal gingiva
- 1: Mild inflammation, slight color change, slight edema, and no bleeding on
probing
- 2: Moderate inflammation, redness, edema, glazing, and bleeding on probing
- 3: Severe inflammation, marked redness, edema, ulceration, and spontaneous bleeding

Q: What is the modified Gingival Index?

Following is the modified Gingival Index:

- 0: Absence of inflammation
- 1: Mild inflammation, slight color change, and slight edema but not involving the entire marginal or papillary unit and no bleeding on probing
- 2: Mild inflammation, slight color change, and slight edema involving the entire marginal or papillary unit and no bleeding on probing
- 3: Moderate inflammation, redness, edema, glazing, bleeding on probing, and hypertrophy of the entire marginal unit
- 4: Severe inflammation

Q: How early can bleeding on probing occur?

Bleeding on probing can occur as early as 2 days after gingivitis begins.

Q: Describe the Periodontal Index.

In the Periodontal Index (Russell[13]), the supporting tissues around the tooth are scored. Periodontal probing is not recommended.

- 0: Negative
- 1: Mild inflammation
- 2: Gingivitis
- 6: Gingivitis with pocket formation
- 8: Advanced destruction with loss of masticatory function

Q: What is the Periodontal Disease Index? What teeth are used in the index?

The teeth used in the Periodontal Disease Index (Ramfjord[14]) are the maxillary right first molar, left central incisor, and first premolar as well as the mandibular left first molar, right central incisor, and first premolar. The cementoenamel junction is used as the fixed landmark to measure periodontal attachment loss.

- G0: Absence of disease
- G1: Mild to moderate inflammation not extending around the tooth
- G2: Mild to moderate inflammation extending around the tooth
- G3: Severe gingivitis and redness

Q: What is the Plaque Index?

The Plaque Index (Löe[12]) is based on the thickness of soft deposits found around a tooth by running a probe along the gingival crevice.

- 0: No plaque
- 1: Film of plaque
- 2: Moderate accumulation of plaque within the gingival pocket or on the tooth and gingival margin that can be seen with the naked eye.
- 3: Abundance of plaque within the gingival pocket or on the tooth and gingival margin.

Prevalence of Periodontitis

Q: What percentage of tooth extractions are caused by periodontitis?

According to Brown et al,[15] 30% to 35% of all tooth extractions are caused by periodontitis.

Q: What percentage of the population has aggressive, chronic, and severe periodontitis?

- Localized aggressive periodontitis: 0.53% (greater prevalence in blacks[7]; many studies have proposed that there may be a defect in neutrophil function)
- Generalized aggressive periodontitis: 0.13%

The 2009 and 2010 National Health and Nutrition Examination Survey[16] found the following data on the prevalence of periodontitis among adults in the United States:

- 47.2% have periodontitis
- 8.7% have mild periodontitis
- 30% have moderate periodontitis
- 8.5% have severe periodontitis
- 64% of adults 65 years of age and older have periodontitis

Association of Periodontitis with Other Conditions

Q: Is there a relationship between periodontitis and preterm births and low birth weight?

A *preterm birth* is defined as one that occurs before 37 weeks gestation; low birth weight is less than 2,500 grams. According to Offenbacher et al,[17] the incidence of preterm birth was 11.2% among women with no periodontal disease and 28.6% in women with moderate to severe periodontitis. However, according to Michalowicz et al,[18] treatment of periodontitis in pregnant women was safe and improved periodontitis, but it did not alter rates of preterm birth. Figure 4-1 presents the current theory of the relationship between periodontitis and preterm birth.

Fig 4-1 Preterm birth and periodontitis. PGE—prostaglandin E_2.

Q: Does food impaction contribute to periodontal pathosis?

Open contacts are correlated with food impaction, and food impaction is correlated with increased probing depth. However, there is no direct relationship between open contacts and increased pocket depth.[19]

Jernberg et al[20] found less plaque but increased probing depth and attachment loss at open contacts.

Q: Do overhanging dental margins contribute to periodontal pathosis?

Overhanging dental margins can be a nidus of periodontal pathogens due to their bulk and roughness and make dental hygiene challenging for the patient and the provider. Pack et al[21] studied 100 patients and found that the percentage of pockets greater than 3 mm was 64.3% among those adjacent to overhanging margins but only 49.2% in pockets neighboring restored surfaces in the absence of overhanging margins and 23.1% in those next to unrestored surfaces.

Brunsvold and Lane[22] found an increase in bleeding, gingivitis, and bone loss in tissues next to overhanging dental margins. They also reported that removal of the overhanging margins improved the effectiveness of hygiene procedures.

Q: Does mouth breathing affect the periodontal tissues?

Mouth breathing can cause dehydration of the gingival tissues, which can result in greater gingivitis in the anterior region. Gulati et al[23] found that in study participants with an incompetent lip seal, the Gingival Index was higher in those who breathed through the mouth compared with those who breathed normally.

Q: Is there an association between malalignment of the teeth and periodontal disease?

With controls for social group and sex, periodontal disease was found more commonly in the maxilla in connection with overjet, crowding, and crossbite. No association was found in the mandible.[24]

Smoking and Periodontal Disease

Q: How does smoking affect periodontitis?

Figure 4-2 presents the relationship of smoking and periodontitis. Smoking increases expression of the cytokines involved in periodontal destruction. Furthermore, the acrolein and acetaldehyde in smoke inhibit human gingival fibroblasts. Lastly, it can cause negative effects on polymorphonuclear leukocytes (PMNs), causing abnormal phagocytosis.

Martins et al[25] found a correlation between failure to cover the root and heavy smoking. Grossi et al[26] found that heavy smokers have six to seven times more alveolar bone loss. It has also been shown that 90% of persons with refractory periodontitis are smokers. Haffajee and Socransky[27] found that smokers have increased bacteria subgingivally.

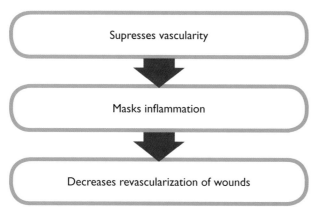

Fig 4-2 How smoking affects periodontitis.

Q: **How should a dentist manage a patient who smokes?**

The dental professional should follow the five As for managing patients who smoke[28]:

1. Ask about smoking at each appointment.
2. Advise and educate the patient on the benefits of quitting.
3. Assess the patient's willingness to quit.
4. Assist the patient with developing a plan to quit.
5. Arrange for follow-up visits.

Q: **Does smoking cessation affect periodontal therapy?**

Kaldahl et al[29] found that a history of smoking did not adversely affect the outcome of therapy: Both past smokers and nonsmokers responded more favorably to therapy compared with heavy and light smokers.

Q: **Is there a difference between smoking a pipe or cigars versus cigarettes?**

In a study on 690 dentate men, Krall et al[30] found an increased risk for tooth loss in men who smoked cigars or pipes and for alveolar bone loss in cigar smokers similar to that observed in cigarette smokers. As a result, the authors recommended that smoking prevention and cessation programs should be targeted to users of all tobacco products.

Biofilms and Plaque

Q: What are some characteristics of biofilms?

Biofilms are dynamic and optimally organized to make use of nutrients. They have greater stability, more cohesiveness, and greater antibiotic resistance compared with their free-living counterparts.

Q: What are plaque and calculus?

Plaque is an organized mass consisting mainly of microorganisms that adhere to the teeth. It consists of bacterial byproducts such as enzymes, food debris, calcium, and phosphate. The organic composition is polysaccharides and proteins, and the inorganic composition is calcium and phosphorus. *Calculus* is made of calcium phosphate salts.

Q: What are the specific and nonspecific plaque hypotheses (Loesche and Giordano[31])?

- Specific plaque hypothesis: Only certain microorganisms cause disease.
- Nonspecific plaque hypothesis: Periodontitis and caries are the result of noxious agents from the entire bacterial population.

Bacteria

Q: Describe the bacteria present in periodontitis.

Table 4-1 presents the properties of bacteria found in periodontitis.

Table 4-1 | Bacteria in periodontitis

Bacteria	Oxygen requirement	Motility	Properties	Virulence factors
Aggregatibacter actinomycetem-comitans	Facultative anaerobe	Nonmotile	- Short, gram-negative rod - Fibroblast inhibiting factor - Lymphocyte suppressing factor - Associated with localized aggressive periodontitis	- Leukotoxin: Kills PMNs and macrophages - Lipopolysaccharide (LPS): Produces collagenase and can induce bone resorption - Hemolytic
Porphyromonas gingivalis	Obligate anaerobe	Nonmotile	- Gram-negative, non–spore forming - Contains porphyrin pigments and fimbriae - *Bacteroides* genus - Associated with advanced periodontal disease	- Gingipains cleave the host proteins between arginine and lysine - Significant hemolytic activity - LPS: Produces collagenase and can induce bone resorption - Inhibits interleukin 8
Prevotella intermedia	Anaerobe	Nonmotile	- Gram-negative, black pigmented - Contain fimbriae - Common in pregnancy because of increased steroid uptake - Common in patients with necrotizing ulcerative gingivitis	- High hemolytic activity - Matrix metalloproteinases destroy the connective tissue - Involved in actin polymerization of the cytoskeleton
Fusobacterium nucleatum	Anaerobe (can grow in 6% oxygen)	Nonmotile	- Gram-negative, non–spore forming, spindle shaped - Principal and frequent bacterial species associated with gingivitis and periodontitis	- Butyric acid: Inhibits fibroblasts and decreases wound healing - Can act as a bridge between otherwise noncoagulating pairs of species - PMN apoptosis - Supports growth of *P gingivalis* in oxygenated or carbon dioxide–depleted environments - LPS: Produces collagenase and can induce bone resorption

Table 4-1 (cont) | Bacteria in periodontitis

Bacteria	Oxygen requirement	Motility	Properties	Virulence factors
Tannerella forsythia	Anaerobe	Nonmotile	- Gram-negative, filament shaped - Found in refractory and advanced periodontitis - Associated with early implant failure	- Contains a surface layer that is believed to delay the host immune response[32] - Trypsin-like protease - Hemolytic activity - Sialidase involved in tissue destruction - Bacterial surface protein A is involved in binding and induces an antibody reaction in periodontal disease[33]
Treponema denticola	Anaerobe	Highly motile	- Spiral shaped - Difficult to study because it is hard to cultivate and slow growing - Found in necrotizing ulcerative gingivitis	- Spore-forming surface protein - Acylated protease complex - Mediates adherence, proteolytic activity, and cytotoxic effects

Q: Describe the red, yellow, orange, and green bacterial complexes first described by Socransky et al[34] in 1998.

Figure 4-3 presents the bacterial complexes. The red complex bacteria increase in prevalence and numbers with increasing pocket depth. Similarly, all species in the orange complex show a significant association with increasing pocket depth as exemplified by *P intermedia* and *F nucleatum*. The remaining complexes showed no statistically significant relationship with pocket depth.

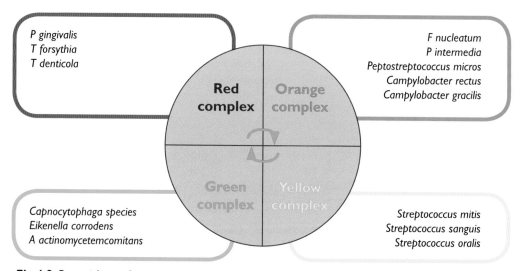

P gingivalis
T forsythia
T denticola

Red complex

Orange complex

F nucleatum
P intermedia
Peptostreptococcus micros
Campylobacter rectus
Campylobacter gracilis

Green complex

Yellow complex

Capnocytophaga species
Eikenella corrodens
A actinomycetemcomitans

Streptococcus mitis
Streptococcus sanguis
Streptococcus oralis

Fig 4-3 Bacterial complexes.

Q: What bacterial changes occur in the transition from health to disease?

Figure 4-4 presents bacterial properties in periodontal health and disease.

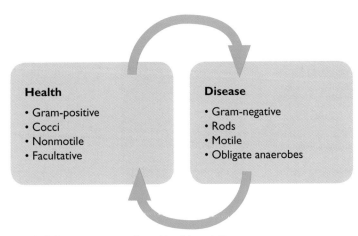

Fig 4-4 Bacteria in periodontal health and disease.

Q: **What percentages of gram-positive and gram-negative bacteria are harbored in gingivitis?**

The bacteria in gingivitis are about 50% gram-positive and 50% gram-negative.

Q: **Which bacteria are associated with health? Gingivitis? Localized aggressive periodontitis? Chronic periodontitis?**

- Health: Bacteria associated with health include *Streptococcus sanguis*, *Streptococcus mitis*, *Actinomyces viscosus*, and *Actinomyces naeslundi*.
- Gingivitis: Lie et al[35] found *Prevotella nigrescens* at the start of gingivitis and after 14 days of experimental gingivitis. Tanner et al[36] studied 56 individuals and found that the predominant species in gingivitis were *A naeslundii*, *Campylobacter gracilis*, and *T forsythia*.
- Aggressive periodontitis: *A actinomycetemcomitans* is associated with localized aggressive periodontitis.
- Chronic periodontitis: *P gingivalis*, *T forsythia*, *F nucleatum*, and *P intermedia* are strongly associated with chronic periodontitis.

Q: **Which bacteria are associated with refractory periodontal disease? HIV/AIDS? Necrotizing periodontal diseases?**

The bacteria associated with refractory periodontitis, HIV/AIDS, and necrotizing periodontal diseases are shown in Fig 4-5.

Refractory periodontitis	HIV/AIDS	Necrotizing periodontal diseases
T forsythia, P intermedia, and P gingivalis	A actinomycetemcomitans and P gingivalis	Spirochetes (T denticola) and P intermedia

Fig 4-5 Bacteria associated with refractory periodontitis, HIV/AIDS, and necrotizing periodontal diseases.

Q: Which bacteria are associated with implant failure? Diabetes? Preterm birth?

- Implant failure: T forsythia, spirochetes, and P gingivalis
- Diabetes: Capnocytophaga species, P gingivalis, and P intermedia
- Preterm birth and low birth weight: A actinomycetemcomitans, P gingivalis, T forsythia, and T denticola

Q: Can bacteria associated with periodontal disease be transmitted from one individual to another?

Offenbacher et al[37] examined 14 married couples to determine the degree of similarity of periodontal flora. They found three times greater odds of observing medium spirochetes and 30% greater odds of the presence of filaments in a patient if the spouse carried the same morphotype. They further stated that, according to their analysis, the presence of these morphotypes in the spouse conferred risk but was not required for the presence of the morphotype in an individual. Asikainen et al[38] found parent-child transmission of A actinomycetemcomitans in 6 of 19 (32%) families. P gingivalis was not transmitted from parent to child in any of the families.

Viruses

Q: Do viruses play any role in periodontal disease?

According to Slots et al,[39] active cytomegalovirus and Epstein-Barr infections have been implicated in the etiopathogenesis of apical periodontitis. In addition, the release of tissue-destructive cytokines, the overgrowth of pathogenic bacteria, and the initiation of cytotoxic or immunopathologic events in periapical pathosis may be caused by herpesviruses.

References

1. Grossi S. Smoking and stress: Common denominators for periodontal disease, heart disease, and diabetes mellitus. Compend Contin Educ Dent Suppl 2000;(30):31–39.
2. Listgarten MA. Pathogenesis of periodontitis. J Clin Periodontol 1986;13:418–430.
3. Löe H, Anerud A, Boysen H, Morrison E. Natural history of periodontal disease in man. Rapid, moderate and no loss of attachment in Sri Lankan laborers 14 to 46 years of age. J Clin Periodontol 1986;13:431–445.
4. Grossi SG, Skrepcinski FB, DeCaro T, et al. Treatment of periodontal disease in diabetics reduces glycated hemoglobin. J Periodontol 1997;68:713–719.
5. Kornman KS, Crane A, Wang HY, et al. The interleukin-1 genotype as a severity factor in adult periodontal disease. J Clin Periodontol 1997;24:72–77.
6. Michalowicz BS, Aeppli D, Virag JG, et al. Periodontal findings in adult twins. J Periodontol 1991;62:293–299.
7. Löe H, Brown LJ. Early onset periodontitis in the United States of America. J Periodontol 1991;62:608–616.
8. Gorman A, Kaye EK, Apovian C, Fung TT, Nunn M, Garcia RI. Overweight and obesity predict time to periodontal disease progression in men. J Clin Periodontol 2012;39:107–114.
9. Shepherd S. Alcohol consumption a risk factor for periodontal disease. Evid Based Dent 2011;12(3):76.
10. Genco RJ, Ho AW, Grossi SG, Dunford RG, Tedesco LA. Relationship of stress, distress and inadequate coping behaviors to periodontal disease. J Periodontol 1999;70:711–723.
11. American Academy of Periodontology. Media Alert: Injectable Progesterone Contraceptives May Be Associated with Poor Periodontal Health. http://www.perio.org/consumer/contraceptives.htm. Accessed 16 September 2012.
12. Löe H. The Gingival Index, the Plaque Index and the Retention Index Systems. J Periodontol 1967;38(6 suppl):610–616.
13. Russell AL. A system of classification and scoring for prevalence surveys of periodontal disease. J Dent Res 1956;35:350–359.
14. Ramfjord SP. The Periodontal Disease Index (PDI). J Periodontol 1967;38(6 suppl):602–610.
15. Brown LJ, Oliver RC, Löe H. Periodontal diseases in the U.S. in 1981: Prevalence, severity, extent, and role in tooth mortality. J Periodontol 1989;60:363–370.
16. Eke PI, Dye BA, Wei L, et al. Prevalence of periodontitis in adults in the United States: 2009 and 2010. J Dent Res 2012;91:914–920.
17. Offenbacher S, Boggess KA, Murtha AP, et al. Progressive periodontal disease and risk of very preterm delivery. Obstet Gynecol 2006;107:29–36.
18. Michalowicz BS, Hodges JS, DiAngelis AJ, et al. Treatment of periodontal disease and the risk of preterm birth. N Engl J Med 2006;355:1885–1894.
19. Hancock EB, Mayo CV, Schwab RR, Wirthlin MR. Influence of interdental contacts on periodontal status. J Periodontol 1980;51:445–449.
20. Jernberg GR, Bakdash MB, Keenan KM. Relationship between proximal tooth open contacts and periodontal disease. J Periodontol 1983;54:529–533.
21. Pack AR, Coxhead LJ, McDonald BW. The prevalence of overhanging margins in posterior amalgam restorations and periodontal consequences. J Clin Periodontol 1990;17:145–152.
22. Brunsvold MA, Lane JJ. The prevalence of overhanging dental restorations and their relationship to periodontal disease. J Clin Periodontol 1990;17:67–72.
23. Gulati MS, Grewal N, Kaur A. A comparative study of effects of mouth breathing and normal breathing on gingival health in children. J Indian Soc Pedod Prev Dent 1998;16(3):72–83.
24. Helm S, Petersen PE. Causal relation between malocclusion and periodontal health. Acta Odontol Scand 1989;47:223–228.
25. Martins AG, Andia DC, Sallum AW, Sallum EA, Casati MZ, Nociti Júnior FH. Smoking may affect root coverage outcome: A prospective clinical study in humans. J Periodontol 2004;75:586–591.

26. Grossi SG, Genco RJ, Machtei EE, et al. Assessment of risk for periodontal disease. II. Risk indicators for alveolar bone loss. J Periodontol 1995;66:23–29.
27. Haffajee AD, Socransky SS. Relationship of cigarette smoking to the subgingival microbiota. J Clin Periodontol 2001;28:377–388.
28. Clerehugh V, Tugnait A, Genco RJ. Periodontology at a Glance. West Sussex, UK: Wiley-Blackwell, 2009:72.
29. Kaldahl WB, Johnson GK, Patil KD, Kalkwarf KL. Levels of cigarette consumption and response to periodontal therapy. J Periodontol 1996;67:675–681.
30. Krall EA, Garvey AJ, Garcia RI. Alveolar bone loss and tooth loss in male cigar and pipe smokers. J Am Dent Assoc 1999;130:57–64.
31. Loesche WJ, Giordano JR. Treatment paradigms in periodontal disease. Compend Contin Educ Dent 1997;18:221–226,228–230,232.
32. Sekot G, Posch G, Messner P, et al. Potential of the *Tannerella forsythia* S-layer to delay the immune response. J Dent Res 2011;90:109–114.
33. Hall LM, Dunford RG, Genco RJ, Sharma A. Levels of serum immunoglobulin G specific to bacterial surface protein A of *Tannerella forsythia* are related to periodontal status. J Periodontol 2012;83:228–234.
34. Socransky SS, Haffajee AD, Cugini MA, Smith C, Kent RL Jr. Microbial complexes in subgingival plaque. J Clin Periodontol 1998;25:134–144.
35. Lie MA, van der Weijden GA, Timmerman MF, Loos BG, van Steenbergen TJ, van der Velden U. Occurrence of *Prevotella intermedia* and *Prevotella nigrescens* in relation to gingivitis and gingival health. J Clin Periodontol 2001;28:189–193.
36. Tanner A, Maiden MF, Macuch PJ, Murray LL, Kent RL Jr. Microbiota of health, gingivitis, and initial periodontitis. J Clin Periodontol 1998;25:85–98.
37. Offenbacher S, Olsvik B, Tonder A. The similarity of periodontal microorganisms between husband and wife cohabitants. Association or transmission? J Periodontol 1985;56:317–323.
38. Asikainen S, Chen C, Slots J. Likelihood of transmitting *Actinobacillus actinomycetemcomitans* and *Porphyromonas gingivalis* in families with periodontitis. Oral Microbiol Immunol 1996;11:387–394.
39. Slots J, Sabeti M, Simon JH. Herpesviruses in periapical pathosis: An etiopathogenic relationship? Oral Surg Oral Med Oral Pathol Oral Radiol Endod 2003;96:327–331.

Pharmacology

Background

Q: What are the United States Food and Drug Administration pharmaceutical pregnancy categories?[1]

- A: Adequate and well-controlled studies in pregnant women have failed to demonstrate a risk to the fetus in the first trimester of pregnancy (and there is no evidence of risk in later trimesters).
- B: Animal reproduction studies have failed to demonstrate a risk to the fetus, but there are no adequate and well-controlled studies in pregnant women.
- C: Animal reproduction studies have shown an adverse effect on the fetus. There are no adequate and well-controlled studies in humans, but the benefits from the use of the drug in pregnant women may be acceptable despite its potential risks.
- D: There is positive evidence of human fetal risk based on adverse reaction data from investigational or marketing experience or studies in humans, but the potential benefits from the use of the drug in pregnant women may be acceptable despite its potential risks.
- X: Studies in animals or humans have demonstrated fetal abnormalities, and there is positive evidence of fetal risk based on adverse reaction reports from investigational or marketing experience, or both, and the risk of the use of the drug in a pregnant woman clearly outweighs any possible benefit.

Q: **Describe the American Society of Anesthesiologists (ASA) classification.**

The ASA physical status classification system is used by clinicians to assess the fitness of patients before surgery. The categories are:

- 1: Normal, healthy patient
- 2: Patient with mild systemic disease
- 3: Patient with severe systemic disease
- 4: Patient with severe systemic disease that is a constant threat to life
- 5: Moribund patient who is not expected to survive without the surgery
- 6: Patient who has been declared brain-dead and whose organs are being removed for donation purposes

Systemic Antibiotics

Q: **When should systemic antibiotics be prescribed in a dental practice?**

- When there is an active infection (eg, acute periodontal abscess)
- As antibiotic prophylaxis
- When placing bone or a membrane in a surgical site[2]
- To treat aggressive periodontitis (*Actinobacillus actinomycetemcomitans* bacteria invades the tissue and cannot be mechanically removed)
- In some cases when surgery is refused by the patient or is contraindicated
- In cases of recurrent or refractory periodontitis due to persistent subgingival pathogens and possibly weakened host resistance[3]

Q: **How should a dentist choose the correct antibiotic to give a patient?**

- Culture and sensitivity
- DNA probe

However, according to the 2003 periodontal workshop,[4] there is limited evidence to suggest that identification of bacteria and determination of susceptibility to antibiotics is helpful in the management of patients who do not respond to therapy.

Q: **Describe the type and spectrum as well as the drug interactions, side effects, and contraindications of the most commonly prescribed antibiotics in dentistry.**

Table 5-1 presents the antibiotics commonly prescribed in dentistry.

Table 5-1 | Commonly prescribed antibiotics in dentistry

Antibiotic	Type	Spectrum	Drug interactions, side effects, and contraindications
Tetracycline (minocycline and doxy-cycline)	Bacteriostatic	Broad: Many gram-positive and gram-negative bacteria, including anaerobes, rickettsiae, chlamydiae, mycoplasmas[5], and some protozoa (amoebas)	- Should not be taken with warfarin. - Patients should not take antacids or consume dairy products. - Birth control pills may become less effective. - Patients with renal dysfunction should not take tetracycline.
Metronidazole	Bactericidal	Obligate anaerobes, *Porphyromonas gingivalis*, *Prevotella intermedia*; also treats acute necrotizing ulcerative gingivitis	- Patients should not consume alcohol. - May increase the effect of warfarin.
Amoxicillin	Bactericidal	Broad: Kills many gram-negative anaerobes and gram-positive bacteria	- Can make birth control pills less effective.
Clindamycin	Bacteriostatic	Aerobic gram-negative and gram-positive cocci; anaerobic gram-negative rod-shaped bacteria, including some bacteroides, fusobacterium, and *Prevotella* species, although resistance is increasing in *Bacteroides fragilis*	- May cause pseudomembranous colitis. - Do not use in kidney transplant patients.
Amoxicillin and metronidazole	Bactericidal	Broad: Used for treating patients with localized aggressive periodontitis	- Patients should not consume alcohol. - May increase the effect of warfarin. - Can make birth control pills less effective.

Q: **What is the dosage for each antibiotic?**

- Metronidazole and amoxicillin: 250 to 500 mg three times a day for 8 days
- Amoxicillin: 250 to 500 mg three times a day for 7 days
- Clindamycin: 300 mg three times a day for 8 days for advanced periodontitis
- Metronidazole: 500 mg three times a day for 8 days for advanced periodontitis
- Augmentin: 500 mg three times a day for 7 days

Q: **What is the effect of systemically administered anti-biotics on clinical measures of attachment level in patients with periodontitis as compared with controls?**

According to a systematic review by Haffajee et al,[6] one can expect about a 0.5-mm improvement in attachment level with scaling and root planing (SRP). They reported greater improvement in clinical attachment levels when systemically administered adjunctive antibiotics were used with and without SRP and/or surgery compared with treatment that did not include their use.

Sgolastra et al[7] demonstrated that full-mouth SRP in addition to systemic use of amoxicillin and metronidazole treatment was effective therapy in patients with generalized aggressive periodontitis.

Lopez et al[8] studied the effect of metronidazole plus amoxicillin as the sole therapy for chronic periodontitis. Twenty-two patients with untreated chronic periodontitis were randomly assigned to a group that received systemically administered 250 mg metronidazole plus 500 mg amoxicillin three times a day for 7 days or to a group receiving SRP and two placebos. The study found similar changes in clinical and microbiologic parameters in both groups. However, there is still insufficient evidence supporting the use of systemic antibiotics as a monotherapy and regarding optimal dosage and duration of systemic antibiotics.

Casarin et al[9] also did a study on metronidazole and amoxicillin and found that the regimen decreased pocket depth and the amount of *A actinomycetemcomitans* when performing full-mouth ultrasonic debridement in generalized aggressive periodontitis patients.

Q: **Which patients need antibiotic prophylaxis?**

Antibiotic prophylaxis is required for:

1. Patients with heart conditions
The American Heart Association[10] recommends the use of preventive antibiotics before certain dental procedures for people with:

- Artificial heart valves
- A history of infective endocarditis
- A cardiac transplant that develops a heart valve problem
- The following congenital (ie, present from birth) heart conditions:
  - Unrepaired or incompletely repaired cyanotic congenital heart disease, including those with palliative shunts and conduits
  - A completely repaired congenital heart defect with a prosthetic material or device, whether placed by surgery or by catheter intervention, during the first 6 months after the procedure
  - Any repaired congenital heart defect with a residual defect at the site or adjacent to the site of a prosthetic patch or a prosthetic device

Prophylactic antibiotics were formerly but are no longer recommended for certain patients, including those with: mitral valve prolapse, rheumatic heart disease, bicuspid valve disease, calcified aortic stenosis, and congenital (ie, present from birth) heart conditions such as ventricular septal defect, atrial septal defect, and hypertrophic cardiomyopathy.

2. Patients with joint replacement

Given the potential adverse outcomes and cost of treating an infected joint replacement, the American Academy of Orthopaedic Surgeons[11] recommends that clinicians consider antibiotic prophylaxis prior to any invasive procedure that may cause bacteremia for joint replacement patients with one or more of the following risk factors:

- Prosthetic joint replacement
- Immunocompromise/immunosuppression
- Inflammatory arthropathies (eg, rheumatoid arthritis, systemic lupus erythematosus)
- Drug-induced immunosuppression
- Radiation-induced immunosuppression
- Patients with comorbidities (eg, diabetes, obesity, HIV, smoking)
- Previous prosthetic joint infections
- Malnourishment
- Hemophilia
- Insulin-dependent (type 1) diabetes
- Malignancy
- Megaprostheses

Q: What is the regimen for antibiotic prophylaxis?

According to the American Dental Association (ADA),[12] the suggested antibiotic regimen is as follows:

- Patients not allergic to penicillin: Cephalexin, cephradine, or amoxicillin 2 g orally 1 hour prior to the dental procedure
- Patients not allergic to penicillin, cefazolin, or ampicillin and unable to take oral medications: Cefazolin 1 g or ampicillin 2 g intramuscularly or intravenously (IV) 1 hour prior to the dental procedure
- Patients allergic to penicillin: Clindamycin 600 mg orally 1 hour prior to the dental procedure
- Patients allergic to penicillin and unable to take oral medications: Clindamycin 600 mg IV 1 hour prior to the dental procedure

Locally Delivered Antibiotics

Q: **What are locally delivered antibiotics?**

Locally delivered antibiotics are those placed in a periodontal pocket with a delivery system and released in a controlled manner, allowing minimum inhibitory concentration for 7 days.

Q: **What are the indications for the use of locally delivered antibiotic therapy?**

The indication for the use of locally delivered antibiotic therapy is when local sites with inflammation have not responded to periodontal or maintenance therapy.

Q: **List the common locally delivered antibiotics and their properties.**

Figure 5-1 presents the properties of the common locally delivered antibiotics.

Actisite (Procter & Gamble/Alza)	Atridox (Atrix)	PerioChip (PerioChip)	Arestin (OraPharma)
• Tetracycline fiber. • Jeffcoat et al[13] found that the adjunctive use of the chlorhexidine chip results in a significant reduction of probing depth when compared with both SRP alone and the adjunctive use of a placebo chip. The chlorhexidine chip is a safe and effective adjunctive chemotherapy for the treatment of adult periodontitis. • This product is no longer available.	• Doxycycline gel 10%. • Bioabsorbable mixture in a syringe. • Placed below the gingival margin, it flows to the bottom of the pocket and adapts to root morphology. • Controlled release over a period of 21 days. • The 2003 workshop on periodontics[14] found a statistically significant improvement in clinical attachment level (CAL) with adjunctive use of the chlorhexidine chip and the doxycycline gel combined with SRP.	• Chlorhexidine chip, 2.5 mg. • The 2003 workshop on periodontics[14] found a statistically significant improvement in CAL with adjunctive use of the chlorhexidine chip and the doxycycline gel combined with SRP.	• Minocycline microsphere (MM) 1 mg. • Bioabsorbable powder. • Grossi et al[15] found that, compared with SRP alone, MM combined with SRP significantly reduced red complex bacteria (RCB) in current smokers and caused a greater improvement in probing depth, bleeding on probing, and CAL regardless of smoking status.

Fig 5-1 Common locally delivered antibiotics and their properties.

Host Modulation

Q: What is host modulation?

Host modulation is adjusting the host response to a microbial challenge.

Q: List the host modulatory products used in periodontics and their properties and related research findings.

Table 5-2 presents the properties and research findings related to host modulatory products used in periodontics.

Table 5-2 | Host modulatory products used in periodontics

Product	Properties	Studies
Subantimicrobial dose doxycycline (SDD) (Periostat, CollaGenex)	- 20 mg doxycycline taken two times a day for 6 to 9 months - Adjunct to conventional treatment in management of chronic periodontitis - No antibacterial activity, but its low concentration blocks enzyme (matrix metalloproteinase) activity involved in tissue destruction	Preshaw et al[16] studied 266 patients over 9 months and found that patients who had SRP and SDD (40 mg) had significantly greater clinical benefits than those with SRP alone in the treatment of periodontitis. In deep sites at month 9, mean CAL gains from baseline were 19% greater with adjunctive once-daily 40-mg SDD than with placebo (2.62 mm versus 2.20 mm, respectively; $P < 0.01$).
Nonsteriodal anti-inflammatory drugs (NSAIDs)	Inhibit prostaglandins	Evidence shows promise that the use of NSAIDS can slow bone loss in chronic periodontitis. However, the safety profile does not support long-term ingestion due to potentially significant side effects.
Bisphosphonates	Inhibit osteoclasts and decrease bone turnover	Reddy et al[17] found that there is a potential role for these agents in periodontitis management.

Bisphosphonates

Q: What is currently known about the risk of periodontal surgery while patients are on bisphosphonate therapy? What is the CTX test and is it reliable?

Bisphosphonates are nonbiodegradable analogs of pyrophosphate with a high affinity for calcium, and they inhibit osteoclasts, thus decreasing bone turnover. Osteonecrosis can result from temporary or permanent loss of blood to the bone. Patients undergoing periodontal surgery who are taking bisphosphonates (especially IV bisphosphonates) have a higher risk of osteonecrosis following surgery.

In a study of 30 patients with osteonecrosis, Marx et al[18] found alendronate (Fosamax, Merck) to be related to a higher incidence of the disease, which had a 94.7% predilection for the posterior mandible and a 50% (15 patients) spontaneous occurrence. The remaining 15 patients had osteonecrosis resulting from an oral surgical procedure, primarily extractions. There was a direct exponential relationship between the size of the exposed bone and the duration of oral bisphosphonate use. About 63% (19/30) of patients reported pain with the bone exposure. The incidence of IV bisphosphonate–induced osteonecrosis in women is 70%.

The morning fasting serum C-terminal telopeptide (CTX; the breakdown product of bone resorption) test correlates to the duration of oral bisphosphonate use and could indicate a recovery of bone remodeling with increased values if the oral bisphosphonate was discontinued. CTX values less than 100 pg/mL represent high risk, between 100 pg/mL and 150 pg/mL represent moderate risk, and above 150 pg/mL represent minimal risk. If CTX values are low, a drug holiday is recommended. In 2008, the ADA released a statement that its expert panel could not recommend CTX testing and drug holidays for predicting and mitigating the risk of bisphosphonate-associated osteonecrosis (BAO) until such measures had been supported by well-controlled, randomized clinical trials.[19]

Q: How should a dentist manage a patient on bisphosphonates?

It is best for patients to have all dental procedures (extractions and surgery) done before bisphosphonate therapy. Specific recommendations for oral and IV bisphosphonates follow:

- Oral bisphosphonates: According to the 2009 American Association of Oral and Maxillofacial Surgeons position paper,[20] although the risk of developing BAO with oral bisphosphonates is low, it appears to increase when therapy lasts more than 3 years or in a shorter period with certain comorbidities such as chronic use of corticosteroids. Therefore, they recommended that, systemic conditions permitting, the clinician consider discontinuing the use of oral bisphosphonates for a 3-month period before and after elective invasive dental surgery as a means of reducing the risk of BAO.
- IV bisphosphonates: If conditions permit, initiation of bisphosphonate therapy should be delayed until dental health has been optimized. This should be a collaborative decision by the treating physician, dentist, and other specialists involved in the care of the patient.

Q: What is the treatment if a patient develops BAO?

Table 5-3 presents treatment for patients with different stages of BAO.

Table 5-3 | Treatment of patients with different stages of BAO*

Risk category	Description	Treatment
At risk	No apparent necrotic bone in patients who have been treated with either oral or IV bisphosphonates	- No treatment indicated - Patient education
Stage 0	No clinical evidence of necrotic bone, but nonspecific clinical findings and symptoms	- Systemic management, including use of pain medication and antibiotics
Stage 1	Exposed and necrotic bone in asymptomatic patients without evidence of infection	- Antibacterial mouthrinse - Clinical follow-up on a quarterly basis - Patient education and review of indications for continued bisphosphonate use
Stage 2	Exposed and necrotic bone associated with infection as evidenced by pain and erythema in the region of exposed bone with or without purulent drainage	- Symptomatic treatment with oral antibiotics - Oral antibacterial mouthrinse - Pain control - Superficial debridement to relieve soft tissue irritation
Stage 3	Exposed and necrotic bone in patients with pain, infection, and one or more of the following: exposed and necrotic bone extending beyond the region of alveolar bone (ie, inferior border and ramus in the mandible; maxillary sinus and zygoma in the maxilla), resulting in pathologic fracture; extraoral fistula; oroantral/oronasal communication; or osteolysis extending to the inferior border of the mandible or the sinus floor	- Antibacterial mouthrinse - Antibiotic therapy and pain control - Surgical debridement/resection for longer-term palliation of infection and pain

*Reprinted from Ruggiero et al[20] with permission.

Local Anesthetics

Q: Describe the local anesthetics used in dentistry.

- Bupivacaine (amino acid; Marcaine, Hospira): Most cardiotoxic, highest lipid solubility and anesthetic potency, strongest vasodilator and longest lasting.
- Mepivacaine (amide; Carbocaine, Hospira and Polocaine, Dentsply): Contains no epinephrine.
- Articaine (amide; Septocaine, Septodont): Some controversy regarding whether it can cause paresthesia when a block injection is given.
- Lidocaine (amino acid; Xylocaine, AstraZeneca): Anti-arrhythmic and local anesthetic.

- Procaine (esther; Novocaine, Hospira): Metabolized in the kidney and not the liver.
- Benzocaine (Orajel orabase, Church & Dwight): Topical anesthetic.
- Prilocaine (amide; Citanest, AstraZeneca): In some patients, a metabolite of prilocaine may cause the unusual side effect of methemoglobinemia.

Q: **In what conditions is epinephrine contraindicated?**

- Pheochromocytoma
- Hyperthyroid crisis
- Supraventricular tachycardia
- Uncontrolled hyperthyroidism
- Recent myocardial infarction
- Unstable angina

Oral Sedation

Q: **Describe the oral sedation medications (benzodiazepines) commonly used in dentistry.**

Table 5-4 lists the medications commonly used in dentistry for oral sedation.

Table 5-4 | Oral sedation medications commonly used in dentistry

Drug	Dosage	Properties	Side effects
Lorazepam (Ativan, Wyeth-Ayerst)	I to 4 mg I hour prior to the procedure	- Does not convert to an active metabolite - Half-life is 12 hours - A sedative and anxiolytic - Has potent amnesic effect	- Adverse effects can include severe sedation and hypotension - Effects are increased in combination with other central nervous system depressant drugs
Diazepam (Valium, Roche)	2 to 10 mg I hour prior to the procedure	- Has an active metabolite - Half-life is greater than 20 hours - Used to treat anxiety and insomnia	Side effects include anterograde amnesia, confusion, and sedation
Alprazolam (Xanax, Pfizer)	0.25 to 0.5 mg I hour prior to the procedure	- Short-acting benzodiazepam - Used to treat anxiety and panic disorders - Half-life is I I hours	Adverse effects include change in libido, ataxia, and slurred speech
Triazolam (Halcion, Pfizer)	0.0125 to 0.25 mg I hour prior to the procedure	- Half-life is 1.5 to 5 hours - Possesses hypoxic, amnesic, anxiolytic, sedative, anticonvulsant, and muscle relaxant properties	Side effects include somnolence, dizziness, feeling of lightness, and altered coordination

Nitrous Oxide

Q: **Describe the properties and advantages of nitrous oxide.**

Properties:
• An inorganic gas
• Very low solubility
• An analgesic and a sedative at the concentrations used in dentistry
• Safe, effective, and reliable

Advantages[21]:
• Quick onset of action
• Ability to be titrated for a rapid recovery
• No risk of motor or sensory impairment following administration
• Low cardiovascular and respiratory depression

IV Sedation

Q: **What are the important instructions to communicate to patients about IV sedation?**

• Do not eat or drink 6 to 8 hours prior to IV sedation.
• You must have a ride home; you cannot drive after IV sedation.

Q: **Describe the IV conscious sedation medications commonly used for periodontal procedures.**

Below are the conscious sedation IV medications commonly used for periodontal procedures. It is important to give a test dose (one drop) of any of these medications before administering the recommended dosage to ensure that the patient has no adverse reactions.

Midazolam (Versed, Roche)
• Benzodiazepine
• Metabolized in the liver and water soluble
• Available in 10-mL vials and given 1 mg/mL
• Lacks active metabolites
• Greater amnesia than diazepam but less duration of clinical effects
• Three times as potent as diazepam
• Half-life is 1.8 to 6 hours

Diazepam (Valium)
- Benzodiazepine
- Ceiling dose is 20 mg
- Most patients need 0.6 to 1 mg
- Not water soluble; IV should be run for a period of time before administering
- Needle should not be inserted on the dorsum of the hand because of the risk of venous irritation
- Half-life is 20 to 100 hours

Fentanyl
- Narcotic analgesic
- 100 times more potent than morphine
- 25 to 50 mg
- Half-life is 2.5 minutes

Meperidine (Demerol, Hospira)
- Opioid analgesic
- Ceiling dose is 50 to 100 mg
- Harder to titrate; better for longer procedures
- Must dilute because of strong histamine reaction
- Half-life is 3 to 5 hours

Q: What are the contraindications for benzodiazepines?

- Use of monoamine oxidase (MAO) inhibitors
- Use of Prozac (Eli Lily)
- Narrow angle glaucoma
- Myasthenia gravis
- Bronchospasm

Q: What medication is given for a benzodiazepine overdose? Opioid overdose?

- Benzodiazepine overdose: Flumazenil is given 0.2 mg/mL; most patients need 0.6 to 1 mg. Its half-life is 20 to 80 minutes. It is important to note that the half-life of flumazenil is shorter than the half-life of midazolam. The patient's vitals must be continually monitored.
- Opioid overdose: Naloxone should be diluted to 1 mg/mL and given 0.1 to 0.2 mg IV every 2 to 3 minutes. Maximum dose is 10 mg. Half-life is 1 to 1.5 hours.

Q: What should be in the IV bag?

Dextrose should be used because distilled water could fractionize. Every 15 drops emitted is approximately 1 mL.

Q: What are some complications that can result from IV sedation?

Figure 5-2 presents the possible complications associated with IV sedation.

Fig 5-2 Possible complications associated with IV sedation.

Pain Relievers

Q: What medications are given for pain?

- Tylenol #3 (McNeil; acetaminophen 300 mg, codeine 30 mg): One tablet every 8 hours
- Vicoprofen (Abbott; hydrocodone 7.5 mg, ibuprofren 200 mg): One tablet every 6 hours
- Vicodin (Abbott; hydrocodone 5 mg, acetaminophen 500 mg): One tablet every 6 hours
- Percocet 5 mg (Endo; oxycodone 5 mg, acetaminophen 325 mg): One tablet every 6 hours
- Percodan (Endo; oxycodone 4.88 mg, aspirin 325 mg): One tablet every 6 hours

Side Effects of Medications

Q: What medications can cause gingival enlargement?

Gingival enlargement is associated with the medications listed in Fig 5-3.

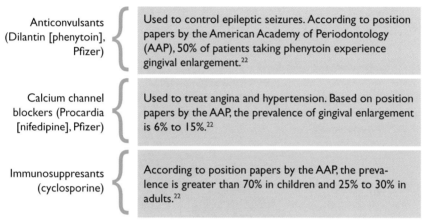

Anticonvulsants (Dilantin [phenytoin], Pfizer)	Used to control epileptic seizures. According to position papers by the American Academy of Periodontology (AAP), 50% of patients taking phenytoin experience gingival enlargement.[22]
Calcium channel blockers (Procardia [nifedipine], Pfizer)	Used to treat angina and hypertension. Based on position papers by the AAP, the prevalence of gingival enlargement is 6% to 15%.[22]
Immunosuppresants (cyclosporine)	According to position papers by the AAP, the prevalence is greater than 70% in children and 25% to 30% in adults.[22]

Fig 5-3 Medications associated with gingival enlargement.

Q: What medications are anti-platelet?

- Plavix (Bristol-Myers Squibb/Sanofi): The patient should not be taken off this medication for routine treatment.
- Aspirin (acetylsalicylic acid): Inhibits thromboxane and cyclooxygenase and interferes with normal platelet function, resulting in prolonged bleeding time.

Q: What medications can cause dry mouth (xerostomia)? What medications can be dispensed to manage dry mouth?

Xanax, Prozac, Lasix (Sanofi Aventis), and antihistamines can cause dry mouth. Radiation and chemotherapy can also contribute to xerostomia.

Biotene gel (GlaxoSmithKline) can be applied to the tongue to relieve dry mouth for up to 8 hours. Another option is Moi-Stir moistening solution (Kingswood Laboratories), which is sprayed directly in the mouth.[23]

Q: What dental conditions are associated with inhalation steroids?

Gingivitis, dental caries, and oral *Candida* are associated with the use of inhalation steroids.

Q: In what situations is it recommended to increase the dosage of a steroid?

Patients with adrenal insufficiency following the use of exogenous glucocorticosteroid hormones are less able to acclimatize to stressful situations. Typically a two- to fourfold increase in glucocorticosteroid dosage on the day of dental treatment will allow the patient to cope with a dental visit. To determine if a patient has adrenal insufficiency, follow the rule of twos[24]:

- A dose of 20 mg or more of cortisone
- For a continuous period of 2 weeks or longer
- In a 2-year time frame

Toothpastes and Mouthrinses

Q: What is triclosan and its mechanism of action?

Triclosan is a phenol nonionic antimicrobial and antifungal agent. Triclosan has the ability to inhibit both the cyclooxygenase and lipoxygenase pathways of arachidonic acid metabolism. As a result, triclosan can inhibit formation of several important mediators of gingival inflammation.

Zambon et al[25] found an association between triclosan and beneficial changes to the bacterial composition of supragingival dental plaque. Colgate Total toothpaste (Colgate-Palmolive) contains triclosan.

Pera et al[26] demonstrated in a double-masked randomized clinical trial that triclosan/copolymer dentifrices allow greater clinical benefits (improved clinical attachment level) following full-mouth debridement in the treatment of generalized severe chronic periodontitis.

Q: What is the spectrum of chlorhexidine (0.12% chlorhexidine gluconate)?

Chlorhexidine is antibacterial (effective on gram-positive and gram-negative bacteria), antifungal, and antiviral. It causes membrane disruption and is found in mouthrinses. It exhibits substantivity, which is the ability to adhere to soft and hard tissues and then be released over time. With continued use, it can cause staining of the teeth, altered taste sensation, and increased supragingival calculus formation.

In a meta-analysis, Gunsolley[27] found seven studies reporting that mouth-rinses with 0.12% chlorhexidine had a strong antiplaque, antigingivitis effect.

Q: What are the active ingredients in Listerine antiseptic rinse and Crest Pro-Health rinse?

- Listerine (McNeil): Methyl salicylate (0.060%) and essential oils (phenolytic compounds, thymol) (0.064%), menthol (0.042%), and eucalyptol (0.092%). The antiplaque efficacy of mouthrinses with essential oils was corroborated by the largest number of studies (21) in the meta-analysis by Gunsolley.[27]
- Crest Pro-Health (Procter & Gamble): Cetylpyridinium chloride (0.07%) (No alcohol).

Q: What are the three major components in toothpaste?

1. Abrasives: Hydrated silica, calcium carbonate, and alumina
2. Therapeutic: Potassium nitrate and sodium fluoride
3. Foaming agents: Sodium lauryl sulfate and hydrogen peroxide

Q: What is the active ingredient in Prevident? Sensodyne?

- Prevident (Colgate-Palmolive): Sodium fluoride 1.1%
- Sensodyne (GlaxoSmithKline): Potassium nitrate 5% and sodium fluoride 0.15%

Miscellaneous

Q: What prescription would a dentist write for a patient with oral *Candida*?

The patient should take 1 teaspoon nystatin 300 mL and rinse for 2 minutes four times a day. Another option is Mycelex troches (Bayer), 10 mg given four times per day for 10 days (dissolves in 30 minutes). It should be noted that Mycelex troches contain sucrose and therefore are associated with a risk of caries.

Q: What medication is prescribed for a patient with an oral viral infection?

The following medications are prescribed for patients with oral viral infections[23]:

- Topical: Acyclovir ointment 5%, 15 g. Patient should be instructed to apply a thin layer to the lesion six times a day for 7 days.
- Systemic: Acyclovir 200 mg, 70 tablets. Patient should be instructed to take one capsule every 4 hours for 2 weeks (maximum of five tablets a day).

References

1. Food and Drug Administration, Department of Health and Human Services. Content and Format for Labeling Human Prescription Drug and Biological Products; Requirements for Pregnancy and Lactation Labeling. http://edocket.access.gpo.gov/2008/pdf/E8-11806.pdf. Accessed 18 September 2012.
2. Sanders JJ, Sepe WW, Bowers GM, et al. Clinical evaluation of freeze-dried bone allografts in periodontal osseous defects. Part III. Composite freeze-dried bone allografts with and without autogenous bone grafts. J Periodontol 1983;54:1–8.
3. Slots J; Research, Science and Therapy Committee. Systemic antibiotics in periodontics. J Periodontol 2004;75:1553–1565.
4. Listgarten MA, Loomer PM. Microbial identification in the management of periodontal diseases. A systematic review. Ann Peridontol 2003;8:182–192.
5. Eliopoulos GM, Roberts MC. Tetracycline therapy: Update. Clin Infect Dis 2003;36:462–467.
6. Haffajee AD, Socransky SS, Gunsolley JC. Systemic anti-infective periodontal therapy. A systematic review. Ann Periodontol 2003;8:115–181.
7. Sgolastra F, Petrucci A, Gatto R, Monaco A. Effectiveness of systemic amoxicillin/metronidazole as an adjunctive therapy to full-mouth scaling and root planing in the treatment of chronic periodontitis: A systematic review and meta-analysis. J Periodontol 2012;83:731–743.
8. López NJ, Socransky SS, Da Silva I, Japlit MR, Haffajee AD. Effects of metronidazole plus amoxicillin as the only therapy on the microbiological and clinical parameters of untreated chronic periodontitis. J Clin Periodontol 2006;33:648–660.
9. Casarin RC, Peloso Ribeiro ED, Sallum EA, Nociti FH Jr, Gonçalves RB, Casati MZ. The combination of amoxicillin and metronidazole improves clinical and microbiologic results of one-stage, full-mouth, ultrasonic debridement in aggressive periodontitis treatment. J Periodontol 2012;83:988–998.
10. American Heart Association. Infective Endocarditis. http://www.heart.org/HEARTORG/Conditions/CongenitalHeartDefects/TheImpactofCongenitalHeartDefects/Infective-Endocarditis_UCM_307108_Article.jsp. Accessed 19 September 2012.
11. American Academy of Orthopaedic Surgeons. Information Statement: Antibiotic Prophylaxis for Bacteremia in Patients with Joint Replacements. http://www.aaos.org/about/papers/advistmt/1033.asp. Accessed 19 September 2012.
12. American Dental Association. Antibiotic Prophylaxis for Dental Patients with Total Joint Replacements. http://www.ada.org/sections/professionalResources/pdfs/ADA_Total_Joint_Replacement_Tables(1).pdf. Accessed 19 September 2012.
13. Jeffcoat MK, Bray KS, Ciancio SG, et al. Adjunctive use of a subgingival controlled-release chlorhexidine chip reduces probing depth and improves attachment level compared with scaling and root planing alone. J Periodontol 1998;69:989–997.
14. Hanes PJ, Purvis JP. Local anti-infective therapy: Pharmacological agents. A systematic review. Ann Periodontol 2003;8:79–98.
15. Grossi SG, Goodson JM, Gunsolley JC, et al. Mechanical therapy with adjunctive minocycline microspheres reduces red-complex bacteria in smokers. J Periodontol 2007;78:1741–1750.
16. Preshaw PM, Novak MJ, Mellonig J, et al. Modified-release subantimicrobial dose doxycycline enhances scaling and root planing in subjects with periodontal disease. J Periodontol 2008;79: 440–452.
17. Reddy MS, Geurs NC, Gunsolley JC. Periodontal host modulation with antiproteinase, anti-inflammatory, and bone-sparing agents. A systematic review. Ann Periodontol 2003;8:12–37.
18. Marx RE, Cillo JE Jr, Ulloa JJ. Oral bisphosphonate-induced osteonecrosis: Risk factors, prediction of risk using serum CTX testing, prevention, and treatment. J Oral Maxillofac Surg 2007;65:2397–2410.

19. Edwards BJ, Hellstein JW, Jacobsen PL, et al. Updated recommendations for managing the care of patients receiving oral bisphosphonate therapy: An advisory statement from the American Dental Association Council on Scientific Affairs. J Am Dent Assoc 2008;139:1674–1677.

20. Ruggiero SL, Dodson TB, Assael LA, et al. American Association of Oral and Maxillofacial Surgeons position paper on bisphosphonate-related osteonecrosis of the jaw—2009 update. Aust Endod J 2009;35:119–130.

21. Newman MG, Takei H, Klokkevold PR, Carranza FA. Carranza's Clinical Periodontology, ed 11. St Louis: Elsevier Saunders, 2012:543.

22. Dongari-Bagtzoglu A; Research, Science and Therapy Committee of the American Academy of Periodontology. Drug-assisted gingival enlargement. J Periodontol 2004;75:1424–1431.

23. Newland JR, Meiller TF, Wynn RL, Crossley HL. Oral Soft Tissue Diseases: A Reference Manual for Diagnosis and Management, ed 2. Hudson, Ohio: Lexi-Comp, 2002.

24. Malamed S. Medical Emergencies in the Dental Office, ed 5. St Louis: Mosby, 2000:149.

25. Zambon JJ, Reynolds HS, Dunford RG, et al. Microbial alterations in supragingival dental plaque in response to a triclosan-containing dentifrice. Oral Microbiol Immunol 1995;10:247–255.

26. Pera C, Ueda P, Casarin RC, et al. Double-masked randomized clinical trial evaluating the effect of a triclosan/copolymer dentifrice on periodontal healing after one-stage full-mouth debridement. J Periodontol 2012;83:909–916.

27. Gunsolley JC. A meta-analysis of six-month studies of antiplaque and antigingivitis agents. J Am Dent Assoc 2006;137:1649–1657.

6

Diagnosis

Background

Q: What is the difference between gingivitis and periodontitis?

Gingivitis is gingival inflammation without loss of connective tissue attachment. *Periodontitis* is gingival inflammation at sites where there has been loss of collagen fibers from cementum and the junctional epithelium has migrated apically. Periodontitis results from the advancement of gingivitis.[1]

Q: What is clinical attachment level?

Clinical attachment level (CAL) is the distance from the cementoenamel junction (CEJ) to the tip of the periodontal probe during normal probing.

Q: What is probing depth?

Probing depth is the distance from the soft tissue margin to the tip of the periodontal probe.

Q: What can affect probing depth?

The following factors may influence probing depth:

- Insertion force
- Size of the probe tip
- Inflammatory status of the tissues

In health, the probe should stop within the junctional epithelium. In patients with periodontitis, it may stop in connective tissue or bone.

Classification

The classification presented in the following answers is taken directly from the 1999 American Academy of Periodontology classification of periodontal diseases.[2]

Q: What are the dental plaque–induced gingival diseases?

I. Gingival diseases
    A. Dental plaque–induced gingival diseases
        1. Gingivitis associated with dental plaque only
            a. without other local contributing factors
            b. with local contributing factors
        2. Gingival diseases modified by systemic factors
            a. associated with the endocrine system
                1) puberty-associated gingivitis
                2) menstrual cycle–associated gingivitis
                3) pregnancy-associated
                    a) gingivitis
                    b) pyogenic granuloma
                4) diabetes mellitus–associated gingivitis
            b. associated with blood dyscrasias
                5) leukemia-associated gingivitis
                6) other
        3. Gingival diseases modified by medications
            a. drug-influenced gingival diseases
                1) drug-influenced gingival enlargements (Fig 6-1)
                2) drug-influenced gingivitis
                    a) oral contraceptive–associated gingivitis
                    b) other
        4. Gingival diseases modified by malnutrition
            a. ascorbic acid–deficiency gingivitis
            b. other

Fig 6-1 Drug-induced gingival enlargement.

Q: What are the non–plaque-induced gingival diseases?

B. Non–plaque-induced gingival lesions
1. Gingival diseases of specific bacterial origin
   a. *Neisseria gonorrhea*–associated lesions
   b. *Treponema pallidum*–associated lesions
   c. streptococcal species–associated lesions
   d. other
2. Gingival diseases of viral origin
   a. herpesvirus infections
      1) primary herpetic gingivostomatitis
      2) recurrent oral herpes
      3) varicella-zoster infections
      4) other
J. Gingival diseases of fungal origin
   a. *Candida* species infections
      1) generalized gingival candidosis
   b. linear gingival erythema
   c. histoplasmosis
   d. other
4. Gingival lesions of genetic origin
   a. hereditary gingival fibromatosis
   b. other
5. Gingival manifestations of systemic conditions
   a. mucocutaneous disorders
      1) lichen planus
      2) pemphigoid
      3) pemphigus vulgaris
      4) erythema multiforme
      5) lupus erythematosus
      6) drug-induced
      7) other
   b. allergic reactions
      1) dental restorative materials
         a) mercury
         b) nickel
         c) acrylic
         d) other
      2) reactions attributed to
         a) toothpaste/dentifrices
         b) mouthrinses/mouthwashes
         c) chewing gum additives
      3) other

6. Traumatic lesions
   a. chemical injury
   b. physical injury
   c. thermal injury
7. Foreign body reactions
8. Not otherwise specified

Q: **What are the two subclassifications for chronic and aggressive periodontitis and their associated extent and severity?**

II. Chronic periodontitis
  A. Localized
  B. Generalized
III. Aggressive periodontitis
  A. Localized (Fig 6-2)
  B. Generalized

    Extent: *Localized* means ≤ 30% of sites are involved and *generalized* means > 30% of sites are involved.
    Severity (based on CAL): Slight = 1 to 2 mm; moderate = 3 to 4 mm; severe ≥ 5 mm.

Fig 6-2 Radiographic appearance of localized aggressive periodontitis.

Q: **How is localized aggressive periodontitis distinguished from generalized aggressive periodontitis?**

Table 6-1 presents the distinguishing characteristics of localized and generalized aggressive periodontitis.

Table 6-1 Localized and generalized aggressive periodontitis*

	Localized aggressive periodontitis	Generalized aggressive periodontitis
Amount of plaque and calculus	Absence of large accumulations of plaque and calculus	Marked periodontal inflammation and heavy accumulations of plaque and calculus
Teeth affected	Interproximal attachment loss on at least two permanent first molars and incisors, with attachment loss on no more than two teeth other than first molars and incisors	Generalized interproximal attachment loss including at least three teeth that are not first molars and incisors
Population	Occurs in children and adolescents without clinical evidence of systemic disease and is characterized by the severe loss of alveolar bone around permanent teeth	Often considered to be a disease of adolescents and young adults; can begin at any age and often affects the entire dentition
Bacteria involved	*Aggregatibacter actinomycetemcomitans*	*Porphyromonas gingivalis* and *Treponema denticola*

*Based on Califano et al.[3]

Q: How should aggressive periodontitis be treated?

According to most authors, surgical or nonsurgical root debridement should be used in combination with antimicrobial (ie, antibiotic) therapy to treat aggressive periodontitis.[3]

Q: Describe the classification of periodontitis as a manifestation of systemic diseases.

IV. Periodontitis as a manifestation of systemic diseases
    A. Associated with hematologic disorders
      1. Acquired neutropenia
      2. Leukemias
      3. Other

B. Associated with genetic disorders
  1. Familial and cyclic neutropenia
  2. Down syndrome
  3. Leukocyte adhesion deficiency syndrome
  4. Papillon-Lefèvre syndrome
  5. Chediak-Higashi syndrome
  6. Histocytosis syndrome
  7. Glycogen storage disease
  8. Infantile genetic agranulocytosis
  9. Cohen syndrome
  10. Ehlers-Danlos syndrome
  11. Hypophosphatasia
  12. Other
C. Not otherwise specified

Q: **Describe Papillon-Lefèvre syndrome.**

Papillon-Lefèvre syndrome is an autosomal recessive syndrome characterized by hyperkeratosis of the soles of the feet, palms, knees, and elbows. Most patients also have severe periodontitis that leads to early loss of primary and permanent teeth. Neutrophil dysfunction is believed to be the cause of the disease.[4]

Q: **What is the classification system for necrotizing periodontal diseases, abscesses of the periodontium, and periodontitis associated with endodontic lesions?**

I. Necrotizing periodontal diseases
  A. Necrotizing ulcerative gingivitis (NUG)
  B. Necrotizing ulcerative periodontitis (NUP)
II. Abscesses of the periodontium
  A. Gingival abscess
  B. Periodontal   abscess (Fig 6-3)
  C. Pericoronal abscess
    1. Periodontitis associated with endodontic lesions
  D. Combined periodontal-endodontic lesions

Fig 6-3 Periodontal abscess.

Q: What is the classification for the developmental or acquired deformities and conditions?

I. Developmental or acquired deformities and conditions
  A. Localized tooth-related factors that modify or predispose to plaque-induced gingival diseases/periodontitis
   1. Tooth anatomical factors
   2. Dental restorations/appliances
   3. Root fractures
   4. Cervical root resorption and cemental tears
  B. Mucogingival deformities and conditions around teeth
   1 Gingival/soft tissue recession
    a. Facial or lingual surfaces (Fig 6-4)
    b. Interproximal (papillary)
   2. Lack of keratinized gingiva
   3. Decreased vestibular depth
   4. Aberrant frenum/muscle position
   5. Gingival excess
    a. pseudopocket
    b. inconsistent gingival margin
    c. excessive gingival display
    d. gingival enlargement
   6. Abnormal color

Fig 6-4 Gingival soft tissue recession of the facial surfaces causing a mucogingival deformity around the teeth.

  C. Mucogingival deformities and conditions on edentulous ridges
   1. Vertical and/or horizontal ridge deficiency
   2. Lack of gingiva/keratinized tissue
   3. Gingival/soft tissue enlargement
   4. Aberrant frenum/muscle position
   5. Decreased vestibular depth
   6. Abnormal color
  D. Occlusal trauma
   1. Primary occlusal trauma
   2. Secondary occlusal trauma

Q: **What is the classification system that the AAP has developed for periodontal diseases (mostly for insurance purposes)?**

- Case Type I: Gingivitis
- Case Type II: Early periodontitis–Mild bone loss with no furcation invasion
- Case Type III: Moderate periodontitis–Moderate bone loss with early furcation invasion
- Case Type IV: Advanced periodontitis–Severe bone loss with far-reaching furcation invasion

Predictors of Diagnosis

Q: **Is bleeding on probing (BOP) a reliable predictor of periodontal disease progression?**

The following studies investigated the reliability of BOP as a predictor of periodontal disease progression:

- Lang et al[5] evaluated 41 patients using BOP at each maintenance visit and found a 6% positive predictive value and a 98% negative predictive value for disease progression. They concluded that BOP is a reliable predictor of periodontal health maintenance.
- Lang et al[6] conducted a retrospective study to evaluate the prognostic value of BOP in identifying sites at risk for periodontal breakdown during the maintenance phase of periodontal therapy. Pockets with an incidence of BOP of 4/4 had a 30% chance of losing attachment. As BOP decreased, the chance of attachment loss also decreased: BOP of 3/4—14%, 2/4—6%, 1/4—3%, and 0/4—1.5%.
- A study by Greenstein et al[7] found that while both inflammation and BOP could be used to identify gingival inflammatory lesions, in areas where observation of inflammatory signs was not possible, BOP using controlled pressure on insertion served as an objective method of diagnosis of inflammatory lesions.
- Haffajee et al[8] evaluated the sensitivity of clinical measurements of gingival redness, plaque, suppuration, and BOP. Because no clinical parameter demonstrated high sensitivity and high specificity values, none of the clinical parameters used individually or in combination were found useful in predicting disease activity at individual sites.

Q: How much pressure should be applied to a probe when measuring BOP?

According to Gerber et al,[9] false-positive BOP results around teeth could be minimized by using a probing pressure of 0.25 N, and around implants a threshold pressure of 0.15 N could reduce false positives.

Q: Is suppuration a predictor of periodontal disease?

Suppuration is found in 3% to 5% of sites with periodontal disease.

Q: Are clinical attachment loss measurements, the distance from the CEJ to the base of the probeable crevice, a good predictor of periodontal disease?

Clinical attachment loss is difficult to accurately measure, but it gives a better overall estimate of the amount of damage to the periodontium than do pocket depth measurements. In prospective studies, clinical attachment loss measurements are the most valid method of assessing treatment outcomes.[1]

Q: Is pocket depth a good predictor of periodontal disease?

In terms of disease progression, Isidor et al[10] found a low positive predictive value for deep probing depth but a very high negative predictive value for absence of pocket depth.

Armitage et al[11] concluded the following from studies in beagle dogs:

- Periodontal probes do not precisely measure connective tissue attachment levels.
- Inflammation has a significant influence on the degree of probe penetration.
- Histologic and clinical sulcus depths differ significantly.

Q: Are there any host-based tests for susceptibility to periodontitis?

There is a test for the interleukin 1 gene cluster available to practitioners. According to the position paper by the AAP,[1] individuals with this composite genotype may have an increased risk of BOP, severe chronic periodontitis, tooth loss, and diminished stability of clinical attachment gain following guided tissue regeneration.

Diagnostic Process

Q: What are some important factors when determining a diagnosis?

The medical history questionnaire and examination are vital and should include the factors[12] listed in Fig 6-5.

| Chief complaint of the patient | History of the complaint | Past and present medical history |

| Drug history | Family history | Extraoral and intraoral examination |

Fig 6-5 Factors to be included in a medical health questionnaire. The medical doctor may need to be contacted to determine if there is a possible dental contraindication.

Q: In which situations are biopsies required?

- A cancerous lesion is suspected
- A positive histologic diagnosis has implications for other body systems
- The lesion being diagnosed has variable clinical histologic features

If in doubt, the dentist should always refer.

Radiographs

Q: What may be some important signs seen in radiographs that suggest periodontal disease?

Radiographic signs of periodontal disease may include:

- Break/fuzziness in lamina dura
- Wedge-shaped radiolucency
- Crestal fuzziness may be an early sign of angular bone loss

Q: Are radiographs an accurate method of diagnosing periodontal disease?

Ortman et al[13] found that the unaided eye is able to detect radiographic changes when approximately 50% of the bone has been lost (Fig 6-6).

Fig 6-6 Radiograph of a patient with bone loss.

Deas et al[14] found that the furcation arrow is an accurate predictor of furcation invasion 70% of the time. However, when furcation invasions are known to be present, the furcation arrow is seen in less than 40% of sites.

Q: What alveolar crest level represents bone loss on a bitewing radiograph?

Hausmann et al[15] suggested that the radiographic threshold for crestal bone loss is greater than 2 mm from the CEJ to the alveolar crest on bitewing radiographs.

Q: Are digital radiographs equivalent to conventional radiographs in revealing bone loss?

Digital radiographs have dose advantages and are able to enhance images. Khocht et al[16] noted that digital radiographs showed a higher number of sites with bone loss than did conventional radiographs. Bruder et al[17] found that digital radiographs saved time, exposed the patient to less radiation (50% to 60%), allowed versatility in viewing the image, and produced no chemical waste.

Q: When should cone beam computed tomography (CBCT) be used?

According to the American Dental Association,[18] "clinicians should perform radiographic imaging, including CBCT, only after professional justification that the potential clinical benefits will outweigh the risks associated with exposure to ionizing radiation. All radiographic examinations should be indicated clinically and justified appropriately."

Abscesses

Q: **How is a periodontal abscess distinguishable from a pulpal abscess?**

Differences between a periodontal and pulpal abscess are shown in Fig 6-7.

Periodontal abscess {
- A pocket is present
- Vital pulp
- Dull pain
- Mobility
- Lateral radiolucency (possible)

Pulpal abscess {
- Large restoration/caries
- May not be a pocket
- Pain may awaken the patient
- Nonvital pulp
- No mobility
- Fistula at the apex

Fig 6-7 How to distinguish between periodontal and pulpal abscesses.

Q: **How can a gingival abscess be distinguished from a periodontal abscess?**

A gingival abscess is more superficial than a periodontal abscess. It is painful and expands rapidly.

Q: **What causes a periodontal abscess and how is it treated?**

The causes and treatment for periodontal abscesses are presented in Fig 6-8.

Causes
- Foreign substance
- Deep inflammation

Treatment
- Drain the abscess
- Pain killers (ibuprofen)
- Possible antibiotics or tooth removal

Fig 6-8 Causes and treatment for periodontal abscesses.

Q: What is a pericoronal abscess?

A pericoronal abscess occurs when the gingiva associated with erupting third molars becomes inflamed. It may occur because of foreign substance entrapment under the gingiva. The pain may spread to the ear or throat and may worsen into Ludwig angina. The treatment includes irrigating the site under anesthesia, antibiotics if there are systemic factors, and extraction if indicated.[19]

Miscellaneous

Q: Is rheumatoid arthritis (RA) a predictor of periodontal disease?

Pischon et al[20] found that study participants with RA had significantly increased periodontal attachment loss and a significant 8.05-fold increased odds of periodontitis compared with control participants. They stated that this association may be only partially accounted for by oral hygiene.

Gleissner et al[21] suggested that patients with long-term active RA present a substantially higher degree of periodontal disease, including loss of teeth, compared with controls.

References

1. Armitage GC; Research, Science and Therapy Committee of the American Academy of Periodontology. Diagnosis of periodontal diseases. J Periodontol 2003;74:1237–1247 [erratum 2004;75:779].
2. Armitage GC. Development of a classification system for periodontal diseases and conditions. Ann Periodontol 1999;4:1–6.
3. Califano JV; Research, Science and Therapy Committee of the American Academy of Periodontology. Position paper: Periodontal diseases of children and adolescents. J Periodontol 2003;74:1696–1704.
4. Van Dyke TE, Taubman MA, Ebersole JL, et al. The Papillon-Lefèvre syndrome: Neutrophil dysfunction with severe periodontal disease. Clin Immunol Immunopathol 1984;31:419–429.
5. Lang NP, Adler R, Joss A, Nyman S. Absence of bleeding on probing. An indicator of periodontal stability. J Clin Periodontol 1990;17:714–721.
6. Lang NP, Joss A, Orsanic T, Gusberti FA, Siegrist BE. Bleeding on probing. A predictor for the progression of periodontal disease? J Clin Periodontol 1986;13:590–596.
7. Greenstein G, Caton J, Polson AM. Histologic characteristics associated with bleeding after probing and visual signs of inflammation. J Periodontol 1981;52:420–425.
8. Haffajee AD, Socransky SS, Goodson JM. Clinical parameters as predictors of destructive periodontal disease activity. J Clin Periodontol 1983;10:257–265.
9. Gerber JA, Tan WC, Balmer TE, Salvi GE, Lang NP. Bleeding on probing and pocket probing depth in relation to probing pressure and mucosal health around oral implants. Clin Oral Implants Res 2009;20:75–78.

10. Isidor F, Karring T, Attström R. Reproducibility of pocket depth and attachment level measurements when using a flexible splint. J Clin Periodontol 1984;11:662–668.
11. Armitage GC, Svanberg GK, Löe H. Microscopic evaluation of clinical measurements of connective tissue attachment levels. J Clin Periodontol 1977;4:173–190.
12. Clerehugh V, Tugnait A, Genco RJ. Periodontology at a Glance. West Sussex, UK: Wiley-Blackwell, 2009:32.
13. Ortman LF, McHenry K, Hausmann E. Relationship between alveolar bone measured by 125I absorptiometry with analysis of standardized radiographs: 2. Bjorn technique. J Periodontol 1982;53:311–314.
14. Deas DE, Moritz AJ, Mealey BL, McDonnell HT, Powell CA. Clinical reliability of the "furcation arrow" as a diagnostic marker. J Periodontol 2006;77:1436–1441.
15. Hausmann E, Allen K, Clerehugh V. What alveolar crest level on a bite-wing radiograph represents bone loss? J Periodontol 1991;62:570–572.
16. Khocht A, Janal M, Harasty L, Chang KM. Comparison of direct digital and conventional intraoral radiographs in detecting alveolar bone loss. J Am Dent Assoc 2003;134:1468–1475.
17. Bruder GA, Casale J, Goren A, Friedman S. Alteration of computer dental radiography images. J Endod 1999;25:275–276.
18. The American Dental Association Council on Scientific Affairs. The use of cone-beam computed tomography in dentistry: An advisory statement from the American Dental Association Council on Scientific Affairs. J Am Dent Assoc 2012;143:899–902.
19. Serio FG, Hawley C. Manual of Clinical Periodontics. Hudson, OH: Lexi-Comp, 2002.
20. Pischon N, Pischon T, Kröger J, et al. Association among rheumatoid arthritis, oral hygiene, and periodontitis. J Periodontol 2008;79:979–986.
21. Gleissner C, Willershausen B, Kaesser U, Bolten WW. The role of risk factors for periodontal disease in patients with rheumatoid arthritis. Eur J Med Res 1998;3:387–392.

Prognosis

Background

Q: What is prognosis?

Prognosis is a forecast of probable outcome of disease based on the experience of a large number of other patients with similar disease progression.

Q: Describe what Hirschfeld and Wasserman[1] and McFall[2] found in their studies on tooth loss over time.

Hirschfeld and Wasserman[1] used three categories to classify the amount of tooth loss that could be expected (Table 7-1). They studied 600 patients over 22 years in which 39% received surgical care. They found a rate of 7.1% overall tooth loss (0.08 teeth per patient per year), and 31% of the teeth that were lost had furcations. Table 7-1 presents a summary of their findings.

McFall[2] studied 100 patients over 19 years in which 63% received surgical care. He found that 9.8% of all surgically treated teeth were lost, and 7.1% of nonsurgically treated teeth were lost. He also found that 56.9% of teeth with furcations were lost. His findings are presented in Table 7-2.

Table 7-1 | Hirschfeld and Wasserman[1] findings on tooth loss over time

Maintenance	Teeth lost (no.)	Population (%)	Teeth lost (%)
Well-maintained	0–3	83.6%	2.6%
Downhill	4–9	12.6%	22.7%
Extreme downhill	10–23	4.2%	55.4%

Table 7-2 | McFall[2] findings on tooth loss over time

Maintenance	Teeth lost (no.)	Population (%)
Well-maintained	0–3	77%
Downhill	4–9	15%
Extreme downhill	10–23	3%

Based on the above studies, the following conclusions can be made:

- Furcation-involved teeth are lost three to five times as often as other teeth.
- Maxillary molars are most often lost, and mandibular canines are more frequently retained.
- Periodontal disease is bilateral and symmetric.
- Periodontal therapy has 87% to 92% tooth retention.

Q: What amount of tooth loss is expected if patients do not comply with a recommended compliance schedule?

Becker et al[3] found the following amount of tooth loss over 5 years. Treated groups received pocket reduction and scaling and root planing in two quadrants.

- 0.36 teeth lost per year for patients who were not treated
- 0.22 teeth lost per year for patients who were treated but not maintained
- 0.11 teeth lost per year for patients who were treated and maintained

Classification

Q: Describe the McGuire[4] classification of prognosis. What categories were considered?

The McGuire[4] classification, based on tooth loss, is presented in Fig 7-1.

Hopeless prognosis	Questionable prognosis	Poor prognosis	Fair prognosis	Good prognosis
One or more of the following:	One or more of the following:	One or more of the following:	One or more of the following:	One or more of the following:
• Inadequate attachment to support the tooth • Grade III or IV furcation involvement • Miller class III mobility • Tooth or teeth cannot be maintained by the professional and/or the patient	• Greater than 50% attachment loss • Grade II or III furcation involvement not accessible for maintenance • Endodontically involved tooth that must be resolved before periodontal treatment • Tooth or teeth not easily maintained by professional and/or patient	• Up to 50% loss has occurred • Grade II furcation with difficult access to the depth and position of the furcation • Greater than Miller class I mobility • Poor crown-to-root ratio • Lack of patient compliance • Presence of systemic factors	• Up to 25% attachment loss measured clinically and radiographically • Grade I furcation allows access for maintenance • Tooth or teeth can be maintained with proper professional and home care • Limited systemic factors	• Etiologic factors can be controlled • Adequate periodontal support • Tooth or teeth can be adequately maintained by the professional and patient • Controlled systemic factors

Fig 7-1 McGuire[4] classification.

A study by McGuire and Nunn[5] showed a 5- to 8-year prediction accuracy of the above classification of 80%. That decreased to 50% or less when the good prognosis category was removed. As a result, assigning prognoses is ineffective for teeth with an initial prognosis of less than good. Although this system was based on tooth loss, critics believed that the status of the remaining teeth is variable and should be based on periodontal stability (clinical attachment level and radiographic bone measurements). Furthermore, tooth extraction is usually performed by the dentist rather than the patient and may be done for other nonperiodontal reasons.

Q: What amount of time is indicated by short- and long-term prognosis?

Short-term prognosis is less than 5 years, and long-term prognosis is considered greater than 5 years. However, Kwok and Caton[6] believed "periodontal prognostication" to be dynamic, suggesting that it should be reevaluated throughout treatment and maintenance.

Q: Describe the prognostic classification by Kwok and Caton.[6]

The Kwok and Caton[6] classification system is based on the probability of disease progression. The four proposed classifications are shown in Fig 7-2.

Hopeless
The tooth must be extracted.

Unfavorable
The periodontal status of the tooth is influenced by local and/or systemic factors that cannot be controlled.

Questionable
The periodontal status of the tooth is influenced by local and/or systemic factors that may or may not be controlled.

Favorable
The periodontal status of the tooth can be stabilized with comprehensive periodontal treatment and periodontal maintenance.

Fig 7-2 Kwok and Caton[6] classification.

They identified the following general factors:

- Amount of patient compliance.
- Cigarette smoking: Smokers have a greater prevalence of periodontal disease and bone loss.
- Diabetes mellitus: Patients with diabetes have a greater prevalence of periodontal disease and attachment loss.
- Other systemic conditions (neutrophil dysfunction, Papillon-Lefèvre syndrome, Down syndrome, and immunologic dysfunctions).

They further identified the following local factors:

- Deep probing depths and attachment loss
- Anatomical plaque-related factors (furcation involvement, enamel pearls, cervical enamel projections, open contacts, crowding, root proximity, and overhanging restorations)
- Trauma from occlusion and parafunctional habits
- Root fractures (Fig 7-3)
- Mobility

Fig 7-3 Hopeless tooth with a vertical root fracture.

Past Periodontitis and Its Effect on Prognosis

Q: **Is there any harm in not extracting hopeless teeth when treating a periodontitis patient?**

DeVore et al[7] studied 17 patients who received open flap debridement with frequent maintenance on retained hopeless teeth. The study found that retained hopeless and periodontally compromised teeth have no effect on the proximal periodontium of adjacent teeth prior to and following periodontal therapy.

Machtei et al[8] studied 145 teeth and concluded that retained hopeless teeth (with severe periodontal breakdown) without periodontal treatment had a negative effect on the adjacent teeth. They found that it was 10 times more likely for the adjacent teeth to have bone loss.

Q: **Does a history of periodontal disease predispose to future disease?**

McGuire and Nunn[9] found a strong association between prognosis and initial probing depth, furcation involvement, and mobility.

Prognosis of Different Diseases and Therapies

Q: **What is the prognosis of a patient with necrotizing ulcerative gingivitis, necrotizing ulcerative periodontitis, and localized aggressive periodontitis?**

- Necrotizing ulcerative gingivitis: Good prognosis with the control of plaque and secondary factors.
- Necrotizing ulcerative periodontitis: Many are immunocompromised; prognosis depends on systemic factors.
- Localized aggressive periodontitis: Good prognosis with treatment.

Q: **What is the prognosis of a tooth that has been diagnosed with a furcation lesion?**

Cobb[10] reported that over a 15-year period, 19% to 57% of teeth with furcation lesions and only 5% to 10% of teeth without furcation lesions were lost.
    Ramfjord et al[11] discovered that 16 of 17 teeth extracted in 5 years during maintenance and following active treatment initially presented with furcation involvement.

Q: Compare the prognosis of implant therapy and endodontic therapy.

It is important to note that there are many variables to consider when reviewing these articles. For example, some of the articles may be comparing surface characteristics of implants that are no longer used.

According to Christensen,[12] there are many factors to consider when comparing the prognosis of implant and endodontic therapy, most of which are listed below:

- Cost: The implant-supported alternative can be twice as expensive as the endodontic alternative, which may influence a patient's decision.
- Coronal breakdown of the tooth: If endodontic therapy is questionable, extraction of the tooth may be a better alternative.
- Type of supporting bone around the tooth: The quality of the bone in the anterior maxilla and mandible is better for implant placement than that in the posterior maxilla.
- The tooth's ability to support a single crown or fixed prosthesis: Questionable nonvital teeth planned for a fixed prosthesis should be replaced with implants.
- Occlusion: Because of increased chewing forces, endodontic and restorative treatment has a questionable prognosis in bruxers and clenchers. Patients who are bruxers and receive implants require a splint and occlusal equilibration.
- Periodontal condition: The periodontal condition of the teeth needs to be addressed before any decision can be made about treatment.
- Patient's perception of treatment: Each treatment should be thoroughly discussed with patients, because how they perceive the psychologic and physiologic trauma associated with different treatment options may greatly influence their decision.
- Overall health: Considerations include smoking and systemic conditions.
- Time needed for treatment: Implant therapy may take longer because of the time needed for implants to osseointegrate.
- Potential esthetic result: If esthetics would be compromised with an implant, retention of the tooth may be a better option.

Iqbal and Kim[13] did a systematic review and found no differences in survival when comparing teeth with treated root canals and single-tooth implants.

Q: What are some considerations to recognize when deciding to save or extract a tooth?

According to Tarnow,[14] the dentist should consider the following:

- Restorative needs of the patient
- Size of the defect
- Endodontic status of the tooth or teeth
- History of periodontal disease
- Decay rate (may be related to the drugs the patient is taking)
- Esthetics in the area
- Anatomical considerations
- Status of the adjacent teeth
- Economic situation of the patient
- Patient's emotions

Figure 7-4 presents factors to consider when deciding whether to extract or save a tooth.[14]

Extract the tooth	• The tooth (with an existing crown) will need a root canal, crown lengthening, a post, and a new crown • Inadequate amount of tooth structure above the crest • A high chance of decay in the mouth • Periodontal surgery will cause esthetic concerns (eg, loss of papilla) • There are grade III or higher furcations
Save the tooth	• Intact arch • No endodontic needs • Restorations are functional • Adequate amount of tooth structure above the crest • Patient has a low decay rate • Patient has no or little periodontal disease • The tooth is not in the esthetic zone • Patient is emotional about keeping the tooth

Fig 7-4 Considerations when deciding to extract or save a tooth.

Q: Is there a correlation between periodontitis and pulpal changes?

Bender and Seltzer[15] found that teeth with restorations or caries and periodontal disease had a higher likelihood of atrophic pulps than teeth with restorations or caries that did not have periodontal disease.

Mazur and Massler[16] studied 106 periodontally involved teeth from patients aged 19 to 70 years of age. The study failed to confirm a correlation between periodontal disease and pulp tissue changes.

Q: Describe the prognosis of implant therapy versus root resection in molars.

Fugazzotto[17] found the lowest success rate (85%) among single implants in second molar positions, while all other implant treatment in molar sites had a success rate of 97.0% to 98.6%. Molars with root resection and molar implants had the highest failure rate when they were single terminal abutments.

Q: Does a fixed partial denture or single implant have a better prognosis?

According to Lindh et al,[18] in the short term (after 1 year), the success rate is 85.7% for fixed partial dentures and 97.2% for implants with single crowns. After 6 to 7 years, the success rate is 93.6% for fixed partial dentures and 97.5% for implants with single crowns.

Q: Can removable partial dentures affect the periodontal status of the patient?

Zlatarić et al[19] found that removable partial dentures do affect the health of the periodontium. There were significant differences in plaque and gingival indices as well as probing depth, mobility, and gingival recession between abutment and nonabutment teeth. It is important for the removable partial denture to be located as far as possible from the gingival margin because its coverage had a negative effect on gingival health.

According to a literature review by Petridis and Hempton,[20] if good periodontal health is established and maintained through oral hygiene measures prior to prosthetic treatment, removable partial dentures do not cause any harm to the periodontium.

References

1. Hirschfeld L, Wasserman B. A long-term survey of tooth loss in 600 treated periodontal patients. J Periodontol 1978;49:225–237.
2. McFall WT Jr. Tooth loss in 100 treated patients with periodontal disease. A long-term study. J Periodontol 1982;53:539–549.
3. Becker W, Becker BE, Berg LE. Periodontal treatment without maintenance. A retrospective study in 44 patients. J Periodontol 1984;55:505–509.
4. McGuire MK. Prognosis versus actual outcome: A long-term survey of 100 treated periodontal patients under maintenance care. J Periodontol 1991;62:51–58.

5. McGuire MK, Nunn ME. Prognosis versus actual outcome. II. The effectiveness of clinical parameters in developing an accurate prognosis. J Periodontol 1996;67:658–665.
6. Kwok V, Caton JG. Commentary: Prognosis revisited: A system for assigning periodontal prognosis. J Periodontol 2007;78:2063–2071.
7. DeVore CH, Beck FM, Horton JE. Retained "hopeless" teeth. Effects on the proximal periodontium of adjacent teeth. J Periodontol 1988;59:647–651.
8. Machtei EE, Zubrey Y, Ben Yehuda A, Soskolne WA. Proximal bone loss adjacent to periodontally "hopeless" teeth with and without extraction. J Periodontol 1989;60:512–515.
9. McGuire MK, Nunn ME. Prognosis versus actual outcome. III. The effectiveness of clinical parameters in accurately predicting tooth survival. J Periodontol 1996;67:666–674.
10. Cobb CM. Non-surgical pocket therapy: Mechanical. Ann Periodontol 1996;1:443–490.
11. Ramfjord SP, Caffesse RG, Morrison EC, et al. Four modalities of periodontal treatment compared over 5 years. J Clin Periodontol 1987;14:445–452.
12. Christensen GJ. Implant therapy versus endodontic therapy. J Am Dent Assoc 2006;137:1440–1443.
13. Iqbal MK, Kim S. For teeth requiring endodontic treatment, what are the differences in outcomes of restored endodontically treated teeth compared to implant-supported restorations? Int J Oral Maxillofac Implants 2007;22(suppl):96–116.
14. Tarnow DP. When to retain the compromised tooth: Point-counterpoint. Presented at the 98th Annual Meeting of the American Academy of Periodontology, Los Angeles, 1 Oct 2012.
15. Bender IB, Seltzer S. The effect of periodontal disease on the pulp. Oral Surg Oral Med Oral Pathol 1972;33:458–474.
16. Mazur B, Massler M. Influence of periodontal disease on the dental pulp. Oral Surg Oral Med Oral Pathol 1964;17:592–603.
17. Fugazzotto PA. A comparison of the success of root resected molars and molar position implants in function in a private practice: Results of up to 15-plus years. J Periodontol 2001;72:1113–1123.
18. Lindh T, Gunne J, Tillberg A, Molin M. A meta-analysis of implants in partial edentulism. Clin Oral Implants Res 1998;9:80–90.
19. Zlatarić DK, Celebić A, Valentić-Peruzović M. The effect of removable partial dentures on periodontal health of abutment and non-abutment teeth. J Periodontol 2002;73:137–144.
20. Petridis H, Hempton TJ. Periodontal considerations in removable partial denture treatment: A review of the literature. Int J Prosthodont 2001;14:164–172.

Occlusion

Background

Q: What is occlusal trauma?

Occlusal trauma is injury resulting in tissue changes within the attachment apparatus as a result of occlusal forces. *Primary occlusal trauma* is injury resulting in tissue changes from excessive occlusal forces applied to a tooth with normal support. *Secondary occlusal trauma* is injury resulting in tissue changes from normal to excessive occlusal forces applied to a tooth or teeth with reduced support.

Q: What are the definitions of abrasion, attrition, and abfraction?

The definitions of *abrasion*, *attrition*, and *abfraction* are provided in Fig 8-1.

> Abrasion: Loss of tooth substance by mechanical wear other than mastication

> Attrition: Occlusal wear from functional contacts with opposing teeth

> Abfraction: Occlusal loading on surfaces causing tooth flexure (in the cervical area)

Fig 8-1 Definitions of *abrasion*, *attrition*, and *abfraction*.

Q: **What are some clinical signs of trauma to the periodontium?**

- Tooth fracture
- Increased tooth mobility
- Loss of the lamina dura and increased periodontal ligament (PDL) space (radiographically)
- Tooth migration
- Pain on chewing
- Occlusal prematurities
- Fremitus
- Hypertrophy of muscles of mastication
- Temporomandibular joint dysfunction

Mobility

Q: **Describe the Miller classification[1] of mobility.**

The Miller classification[1] of mobility:

- Class 1: First sign of movement greater than normal.
- Class 2: The tooth can be moved up to 1 mm in a buccolingual or mesio-distal direction but does not exhibit abnormal mobility in an occlusoapical direction.
- Class 3: The tooth can be moved 1 mm or more in either buccolingual or mesiodistal and occlusoapical directions.

Q: **What are the causes of increased mobility of the teeth?**

- Loss of tooth support
- Trauma from occlusion
- Parafunctional habits
- Short root
- Orthodontic movement
- Extension of inflammation from the gingiva to the PDL
- Periodontal surgery (temporary)
- Pregnancy or menstrual cycle
- Pathologic process

Q: Is there a relationship between mobile teeth and success of periodontal treatment?

Fleszar et al[2] studied 82 patients in 8 years and found that pockets of clinically mobile teeth do not respond as well to periodontal treatment as do those of immobile teeth exhibiting the same initial disease severity.

Grant et al[3] found significantly higher proportions of *Campylobacter rectus* and *Peptostreptococcus micros* in pockets around mobile teeth compared with those adjacent to non-mobile teeth. Elevated levels of *Porphyromonas gingivalis* were also found around mobile teeth, but the difference was not statistically significant. The authors concluded that tooth mobility and its associated increase in subgingival levels of periodontopathogens may present a periodontal risk.

Q: What is fremitus?

Fremitus is a palpable or visible movement of a tooth when it is subjected to occlusal forces.

Types of Occlusion

Q: What is group function? Canine-guided occlusion?

During lateral movement, if there is simultaneous contact of the posterior teeth of the working side, it is called *group function*. In the same situation, if the canine alone contacts, then it is called *canine-guided occlusion* or *canine protection*.

Q: What percent of the population has canine protection? Group function?

Goldstein[4] found that 14% of study participants exhibited canine protection, 46% had group function, and 24% demonstrated a different disocclusion pattern on each side.

Q: What type of occlusion is ideal for patients with implants?

Anterior guidance with no lateral forces on implants is ideal. There should be minimal contact in excursive movements.

Theories of Occlusion

Q: Describe the different theories of occlusion.

- In a cadaver study, Glickman[5] described two regions in the periodontium: the zone of irritation (marginal and interdental gingiva and gingival and transeptal fibers) and the zone of codestruction (PDL, alveolar bone, cementum, and transeptal and alveolar crest fibers). Inflammation of the supporting tissues in the presence of occlusal trauma alters the alignment of the transseptal fibers, allowing inflammation to spread to the PDL space with resultant intrabony pocket formation.
- Based on a cadaver study, Waerhaug[6] believed bacterial plaque in conjunction with local anatomy was the primary cause of intrabony defect formation, not occlusal trauma.
- A study by Lindhe and Svanberg[7] used a jiggling force, applied using a splint cap, on beagle dogs. The study found attachment loss when the bony support was surgically decreased, and inflammation was present with occlusal stress.
- Kennedy and Polson[8] used nonjiggling forces on wooden wedges in squirrel monkeys. They found that trauma caused loss of bone height and a reduction of coronal bone but no loss of attachment.
- Ramfjord and Ash[9] found that traumatic occlusion does not initiate or aggravate gingivitis or initiate pockets, but it can increase mobility and may accelerate bone loss and pocket formation, depending on the presence of inflammation. Bruxism can perpetuate trauma. Splinting is not indicated in self-limiting trauma from occlusion but is indicated in conjunction with occlusal adjustment when trauma from occlusion is progressive.

Occlusal Discrepancies

Q: Do uneven marginal ridges increase attachment loss?

Blieden[10] found that poor contours and marginal discrepancies can increase the risk of periodontal infections.

Kepic and O'Leary[11] did not find increased attachment loss with uneven marginal ridges.

Q: Do teeth with occlusal contacts in excursive positions exhibit any greater severity of periodontitis?

Yuodelis and Mann[12] found that 53% of nonworking contacts had greater pocket depth and greater mobility. However, this study had no controls. Nunn and Harrel[13] found teeth with initial occlusal discrepancies to have significantly deeper initial probing depths, significantly worse prognoses, and significantly worse mobility than teeth without initial occlusal discrepancies.

Pihlstrom et al[14] found that teeth with occlusal contacts in centric relation and working, nonworking, or protrusive positions did not exhibit any greater severity of periodontitis than teeth without these contacts. Shefter and McFall[15] found that nonfunctional contacts are common and that occlusal disharmonies do not have a significant harmful impact on periodontal health.

Q: Do occlusal discrepancies affect gingival recession?

According to Harrel and Nunn,[16] there is no statistically significant relationship between the presence of occlusal discrepancies and initial width of the gingival tissue or between occlusal treatment and changes in the width of the gingiva.

Bruxism

Q: What are symptoms of bruxism?

The symptoms of bruxism include the following[17]:

- Increased mobility
- Pulpal sensitivity
- Bite tenderness
- Excessive occlusal wear
- Muscle tenderness
- Temporomandibular joint pain
- Audible sound

Q: Can periodontal disease be affected by bruxism?

Hanamura et al[18] found significantly greater alveolar bone loss, attachment loss, and tooth mobility in patients with moderate to severe periodontitis than in patients with bruxism, while more tooth attrition was found in the bruxism patients. In most cases, periodontal disease and bruxism did not co-exist in the same individual, and the authors concluded that in general there was no close association between the two conditions.

Occlusal Adjustment

Q: What is occlusal adjustment?

Occlusal adjustment is the grinding of occlusal surfaces of teeth to create a balanced relationship between the maxillary and mandibular teeth. It is important to remove centric prematurities, preserve the supporting cusps, and remove lateral contacts.

Q: What are the indications and contraindications for occlusal adjustment?

Figure 8-2 presents the indications and contraindications for occlusal adjustment. Note that according to Lindhe et al,[19] occlusal adjustment is effective against tooth mobility when mobility is caused by increased width of the PDL.

Indications	Contraindications
In conjunction with restorative treatment, orthodontics, orthognathic surgery, or jaw trauma when indicated	Prophylactic treatment
Parafunctional habits	Severe extrusion of malpositioned teeth
Traumatic injuries	The primary treatment for bruxism
Increased mobility	Emotional state of the patient precludes a satisfactory result

Fig 8-2 Indications and contraindications for occlusal adjustment.

Q: **Is there greater gain of clinical periodontal attachment in patients who received occlusal adjustment compared with those who did not?**

According to Burgett et al,[20] there was a significant gain in attachment of 0.4 mm in patients who received occlusal adjustment. Pocket depth was not affected by occlusal adjustment, and the response to occlusal adjustment was not impacted by initial tooth mobility or periodontal disease severity.

Splinting

Q: **When should splinting be done?**

Splinting should be done[21]:

- Following trauma
- For comfort
- To prevent drifting of the teeth
- To prevent mobility

Q: **What are contraindications to splinting?**

Splinting is contraindicated when[22]:

- The treatment of inflammatory periodontal disease has not been addressed
- Occlusal adjustment to reduce trauma or interferences has not been previously addressed
- The sole objective of splinting is to reduce tooth mobility

Consequences of Occlusal Force

Q: **What are the stages of tissue response to increased occlusal forces?**

- Stage 1: The body tries to repair injury from excessive occlusal force. The area most susceptible to injury is the furcation.
- Stage 2: Repair is constantly occurring in the normal periodontium. Trauma from occlusion stimulates increased reparative activity. The damaged tissues are removed, and new connective tissue cell fibers, bone, and cementum are formed.
- Stage 3: Adaptive remodeling occurs. If the repair process cannot keep up with destruction, the periodontium is remodeled. This results in a thickened PDL and increased vascularization.

Q: What are the consequences of insufficient occlusal forces?

Insufficient occlusal forces can cause inadequate stimulation to the PDL, which consequently thins, leading to atrophy of fibers with the result of reduced bone height.

Orthodontics

Q: How does orthodontics help a periodontal patient?

- Aligns the teeth and helps the patient with oral hygiene
- Can improve osseous defects (decrease amount of resective surgery)
- Can force eruption to align the gingiva
- Can force eruption of a cracked tooth (at least 1:1 crown-to-root ratio)
- Closes open embrasures
- Improves adjacent tooth position before implant placement

Q: What are the risks of orthodontic treatment?

- Recession
- Root resorption (shortened root length)
- Loss of attachment
- Loss of tooth vitality
- Tooth relapse
- Caries

Q: Under what circumstances should extrusion be done?

- Increasing bone height prior to extraction of a hopeless tooth and subsequent implant placement: Amato et al[23] found that forced eruption was able to regenerate 70% of bone and augment the gingiva by 60%.
- Crown lengthening (may still need surgery because the bone moves with the tooth).
- Filling intraosseous defects.
- Leveling and aligning the gingival margin for esthetic harmony.

Q: Can tooth movement into adjacent defects be accomplished successfully?

In a study with a monkey model, Polson et al[24] established that orthodontic tooth movement into intrabony periodontal defects with a reduced but healthy periodontium was not damaging to the connective tissue attachment.

Q: Should orthodontics be used to upright a molar?

 A study by Lang[25] demonstrated a 0.6-mm decrease in pocket depth and a 0.4-mm gain in attachment level following uprighting of mandibular tipped molars in advance of prosthetic treatment. He concluded that this technique was a simple and predictable method that would improve the prognosis of the treated teeth.

 Kessler[26] pointed out the risks of uprighting mesially tipped second molars. Bone loss and furcation involvement may be caused by the uprighting as a periodontal osseous lesion is widened when the tooth is uprighted. A study by Lundgren et al[27] concluded that a mesially tipped molar does not increase the risk for periodontal disease compared with an upright molar and therefore did not support the use of orthodontic uprighting to prevent the initiation or advancement of periodontal disease.

Q: Can orthodontics worsen the prognosis of a patient with periodontitis?

The lack of periodontal support may reduce resistance to unwanted tooth movement (anchorage problems) and can increase the risk of root resorption due to reduced available root surface area and decreased vascularity.[28]

A study of periodontal health during orthodontic treatment by Boyd et al[29] included 20 adults (10 of whom received treatment for generalized periodontitis prior to orthodontic treatment) and 20 adolescents. The study found that during fixed orthodontic treatment:

• No significant increase in loss of attachment occurs in patients with a reduced but healthy periodontium.
• Tooth loss may occur in adults with advanced periodontal disease, including pocket depths > 6 mm or advanced furcation involvements.
• Significantly more plaque accumulation and gingival inflammation can be expected in adolescents than in adults.

References

1. Miller SC. Textbook of Periodontia. Philadelphia: Blakiston, 1938.
2. Fleszar TJ, Knowles JW, Morrison EC, Burgett FG, Nissle RR, Ramfjord SP. Tooth mobility and periodontal therapy. J Clin Periodontol 1980;7:495–505.
3. Grant DA, Grant DA, Flynn MJ, Slots J. Periodontal microbiota of mobile and non-mobile teeth. J Periodontol 1995;66:386–390.
4. Goldstein GR. The relationship of canine-protected occlusion to a periodontal index. J Prosthet Dent 1979;41:277–283.
5. Glickman I. Inflammation and trauma from occlusion. Co-destructive factors in chronic periodontal disease. J Periodontol 1963;34:5–10.
6. Waerhaug J. The infrabony pocket and its relationship to trauma from occlusion and subgingival plaque. J Periodontol 1979;50:355–365.
7. Lindhe J, Svanberg G. Influence of trauma from occlusion on progression of experimental periodontitis in the beagle dog. J Clin Periodontol 1974;1:3–14.
8. Kennedy JE, Polson AM. Experimental marginal periodontitis in squirrel monkeys. J Periodontol 1973;44:140–144.
9. Ramfjord SP, Ash MM Jr. Significance of occlusion in the etiology and treatment of early, moderate, and advanced periodontitis. J Periodontol 1981;52:511–517.
10. Blieden TM. Tooth-related issues. Ann Periodontol 1999;4:91–97.
11. Kepic TJ, O'Leary TJ. Role of marginal ridge relationships as an etiologic factor in periodontal disease. J Periodontol 1978;49:570–575.
12. Yuodelis RA, Mann WV Jr. The prevalence and possible role of nonworking contacts in periodontal disease. Periodontics 1965;3:219–223.
13. Nunn ME, Harrel SK. The effect of occlusal discrepancies on periodontitis. I. Relationship of initial occlusal discrepancies to initial clinical parameters. J Periodontol 2001;72:485–494.
14. Pihlstrom BL, Anderson KA, Aeppli D, Schaffer EM. Association between signs of trauma from occlusion and periodontitis. J Periodontol 1986;57:1–6.
15. Shefter GJ, McFall WT Jr. Occlusal relations and periodontal status in human adults. J Periodontol 1984;55:368–374.
16. Harrel SK, Nunn ME. The effect of occlusal discrepancies on gingival width. J Periodontol 2004;75:98–105.
17. Raigrodski AJ. Cosmetic dentistry: The full mouth fixed rehabilitation of the bruxing patient—Achieving function and esthetics. Available at: http://www.oralhealthgroup.com/news/cosmetic-dentistry-the-full-mouth-fixed-rehabilitation-of-the-bruxing-patient--achieving-function-an/1000145772/. Accessed 19 December 2012.
18. Hanamura H, Houston F, Rylander H, Carlsson GE, Haraldson T, Nyman S. Periodontal status and bruxism. A comparative study of patients with periodontal disease and occlusal parafunctions. J Periodontol 1987;58:173–176.
19. Lindhe J, Nyman S, Ericsson I. Trauma from occlusion: Periodontal tissues. In: Lindhe J, Lang NP, Karring T (eds). Clinical Periodontology and Implant Dentistry, ed 5. Oxford, UK: Blackwell Munksgaard, 2008:359.
20. Burgett FG, Ramfjord SP, Nissle RR, Morrison EC, Charbeneau TD, Caffesse RG. A randomized trial of occlusal adjustment in the treatment of periodontitis patients. J Clin Periodontol 1992;19:381–387.
21. Lemmerman K. Rationale for stabilization. J Periodontol 1976;47:405–411.
22. Rupprecht R. Trauma from occlusion: A review. Available from: http://www.med.navy.mil/sites/navmedmpte/npds/acp/Pages/ClinicalUpdates2004.aspx. Accessed 25 September 2012.
23. Amato F, Mirabella AD, Macca U, Tarnow DP. Implant site development by orthodontic forced extraction: A preliminary study. Int J Oral Maxillofac Implants 2012;27:411–420.
24. Polson A, Caton J, Polson AP, Nyman S, Novak J, Reed B. Periodontal response after tooth movement into intrabony defects. J Periodontol 1984;55:197–202.
25. Lang NP. Preprosthetic straightening of tilted lower molars with reference to the condition of the periodontium [in German]. SSO Schweiz Monatsschr Zahnheilkd 1977;87:560–569.
26. Kessler M. Interrelationships between orthodontics and periodontics. Am J Orthod 1976;70:154–172.
27. Lundgren D, Kurol J, Thorstensson B, Hugoson A. Periodontal conditions around tipped and upright molars in adults. An intra-individual retrospective study. Eur J Orthod 1992;14:449–455.
28. Clerehugh V, Tugnait A, Genco R.J. Periodontology at a Glance. West Sussex, UK: Wiley-Blackwell, 2009:58.
29. Boyd RL, Leggott PJ, Quinn RS, Eakle WS, Chambers D. Periodontal implications of orthodontic treatment in adults with reduced or normal periodontal tissues versus those of adolescents. Am J Orthod Dentofacial Orthop 1989;96:191–198.

Nonsurgical Therapy

Background

Q: What treatment does nonsurgical therapy include?

- Plaque control
- Supra- and subgingival scaling and root planing (SRP)
- Use of chemical agents
- Oral hygiene instruction
- Recontouring defective restorations
- Occlusal therapy

Q: What is scaling?

Scaling is instrumentation of the crown and root surfaces of the teeth to remove plaque, calculus, and staining from the teeth.

Q: What is root planing?

Root planing is a treatment procedure to remove cementum or surface dentin that is rough, impregnated with calculus, or contaminated with toxins or microorganisms.

Q: What are the endpoints to successful root planing therapy?

- Excellent oral hygiene
- Pink and firm gingival tissue
- Pocket depth less than 5 mm
- No bleeding on probing (BOP)
- No calculus detected
- Decreased mobility of the teeth

Effectiveness of Scaling and Root Planing

Q: What studies show the effectiveness of SRP?

- A literature review by Cobb[1] found pocket depth reduction of 1.29 mm and attachment gain of 0.55 mm in 4- to 6-mm pockets and pocket depth reduction of 2.16 mm and attachment gain of 1.79 mm in pockets greater than 7 mm. Stambaugh et al[2] found curette efficacy of 3.73 mm (plaque and calculus–free surface) when SRP was performed by hygienists with the patient under local anesthesia. The instrument limit was 6.21 mm. The average time working on each tooth was 35 minutes.
- Buchanan and Robertson[3] noted that premolars and molars are more difficult to clean without a flap. They found that more than 60% of molar sites had residual calculus.
- Waerhaug[4] found that after SRP was performed, more than 90% of cases had deposits of plaque and calculus remaining in sites with pocket depths greater than 5 mm.

Q: What are some factors that can limit the effectiveness of root planing?

Many anatomical factors can limit the effectiveness of root instrumentation[5]:

- Deep probing depths
- Root concavities
- Furcations

Host response may also limit the effectiveness of root instrumentation:

- Diabetes
- Pregnancy
- Stress
- AIDS
- Immunodeficiencies
- Blood dyscrasias

Q: Is root debridement equally effective in molars and nonmolars?

Loos et al[6] found that, following full-mouth root debridement, more molar furcation sites (25%) lost probing attachment compared with non-molar sites (7%) and molar flat-surface sites (10%).

Q: Are more experienced practitioners more effective at SRP?

Brayer et al[7] showed no difference in the effectiveness of SRP in shallow (1- to 3-mm) pockets based on the experience level of the practitioner or type of procedure. However, In moderate (4- to 6-mm) and deep (greater than 6-mm) periodontal pockets, a significantly higher number of calculus-free root surfaces were produced by practitioners with greater experience, and SRP was more effective when combined with an open flap procedure.

Q: Is open flap or closed flap SRP more effective?

Caffesse et al[8] found that residual calculus was greatest following scaling with no flap (Table 9-1) and at the cementoenamel junction or in association with grooves, fossae, or furcations. No differences were noted between anterior and posterior teeth or between different tooth surfaces.

Table 9-1	Percent of calculus-free surface in different pocket depths following scaling with or without a flap		
Scaling	1- to 3-mm pockets	4- to 6-mm pockets	> 6-mm pockets
Without a flap	86%	43%	32%
With a flap	86%	76%	50%

Lindhe et al[9] monitored patients for 5 years following nonsurgical or surgical therapy. A high frequency of plaque-free tooth surfaces was associated with a lack of evidence of recurrent periodontal disease, whereas patients with a high frequency of surfaces with plaque had additional loss of attachment at a greater rate. Surgical and nonsurgical treatment were shown to be equally effective in sites with an initial pocket depth greater than 3 mm. The authors concluded that the quality of root surface debridement is a more important determinant in the success of periodontal therapy than the type of technique used (surgical versus nonsurgical).

Q: What are the consequences to patients with periodontitis who do not receive treatment?

Goodson et al[10] studied attachment level at two sites on each tooth in 22 untreated subjects with existing periodontal pockets for 1 year. They found no significant changes in 82.8% of the sites, significantly deeper pockets in 5.7% of the sites, and significantly shallower pockets in 11.5% of the sites. About half of the sites with increased pocket depth showed cycles of deepening pockets and spontaneous return to the original depth, suggesting that periodontal disease may be a dynamic condition characterized by periods of exacerbation, remission, and inactivity.

Löe et al[11] did a study on Sri Lankan laborers, who, in the absence of oral hygiene practices, presented with large amounts of plaque, calculus, and staining and widespread gingival inflammation. Using interproximal loss of attachment and rates of tooth loss, the authors identified three subpopulations:

- Individuals (approximately 8%) with rapid progression of periodontal disease
- Individuals with moderate progression of periodontal disease (approximately 81%)
- Individuals with no progression (approximately 11%) of periodontal disease beyond gingivitis

Q: What are the critical probing depths?

Using a split-mouth design, Lindhe et al[12] treated 15 patients with moderately advanced periodontal disease using SRP in combination with a modified Widman flap procedure on one side and SRP only on the contralateral side. The study found the following critical probing depths:

- 2.9 mm: Attachment loss occurred in pockets < 2.9 mm when SRP was performed
- 4.2 mm: Attachment loss occurred in pockets < 4.2 mm if SRP and surgery were performed

Q: Is it more effective to do weekly SRP appointments or a single SRP appointment?

Quirynen et al[13] concluded that the use of antiseptics, as well as the completion of the SRP sessions within a short time frame, seems to have a beneficial effect in the treatment of moderate and severe periodontitis.

Greenstein[14] found that full-mouth therapy could reduce the number of patient visits and facilitate more efficient use of treatment time. In addition, he stated that there did not appear to be any major adverse reactions to full-mouth root planing whether or not it was paired with chemotherapy.

Q: Is removal of the cementum important?

Drisko and Killoy[15] suggested that while "thorough root debridement and planing are desirable treatment goals, not all would agree that complete cementum removal is either possible or desirable, or that the removal of calculus is more important than plaque or endotoxin removal in achieving clinical success."

In his literature review, Cobb[1] found that "given the fact that cementum is known to become contaminated when exposed in a periodontal pocket, the literature remains inconsistent concerning both the possibility or need to remove all cementum, and whether it is more important to remove plaque and calculus than 'diseased' cementum."

Q: How many strokes cause removal of the cementum?

Coldiron et al[16] reported that most teeth in groups treated with 20 to 70 strokes showed complete cementum removal, although fragments of cementum remained on the surface of the root in some sections of teeth from each of these treatment groups.

Ritz et al[17] investigated four methods of instrumentation: hand curette, ultrasonic scaler, air scaler, and fine-grit diamond bur. After 12 working strokes, the ultrasonic scaler removed only an 11.6-µm layer of root substance, while much larger amounts of 93.5 µm (air scaler), 108.9 µm (curette), and 118.7 µm (diamond bur) were removed by the other instruments.

Oral Hygiene

Q: How effective is brushing and flossing?

Graves et al[18] found that brushing decreases BOP by 35%, and additional flossing decreased BOP by 67%. Floss is the most widely used method of interdental cleaning, and the American Dental Association reports that up to 80% of interdental plaque may be removed by this method, resulting in a significantly reduced incidence of caries and prevention of periodontal disease.[19]

Q: What is the Bass technique?

In the *Bass technique*,[20] the bristles of a toothbrush are placed at 45 degrees to the tooth surface at the gingival margin. The bristles of the brush are moved in a back-and-forth motion.

Q: Is there a difference between the types of floss and their efficacy?

In a study that involved 24 dental hygiene students, Carr et al[21] tested four different floss types: waxed, unwaxed, woven, and shred-resistant and reported minimal differences in the efficacy, comfort, and ease of use.

Q: Describe the effectiveness of interdental brushes.

In a single-blind, randomized controlled clinical trial, Jackson et al[22] reported that BOP and probing improved more in the interdental brush group than in the floss group at 6 weeks, and at 12 weeks, significantly greater changes in plaque, papillae level, and probing depths were found in the interdental brush group compared with the floss group.

Tu et al[23] used structural equation modeling to show a greater reduction in pocket depth and BOP with the use of interdental brushing compared with flossing. They attributed this difference primarily to plaque removal efficiency rather than interdental papillae compression.

Q: If complete removal of plaque is not accomplished, how long does it take for gingivitis to develop?

Lang et al[24] found that intervals of 48 hours are compatible with gingival health; however, if intervals between complete removal of plaque exceed 48 hours, gingivitis develops. Plaque first appears on interproximal areas of premolars and last on the facial surfaces of molars and premolars.

Q: Is there a difference between an electric and manual brush?

Robinson et al[25] did a meta-analysis and found that powered toothbrushes with a rotation oscillation action reduce plaque and gingivitis more than manual toothbrushes.

Deery et al[26] did not find a statistically significant difference between the results of use of powered and manual brushes in general; however, they did report significant short- and long-term reduction of plaque and gingivitis with the use of rotation oscillation–powered brushes.

Rapley and Killoy[27] compared a counter-rotational electric toothbrush and a manual toothbrush. The manual group had 30.57% plaque-free interproximal surfaces and the electric group had 53.23% plaque-free interproximal surfaces.

Q: **How often should a toothbrush be replaced?**

Glaze and Wade[28] found that after 10 weeks, significantly less plaque had formed in the participants who replaced their brushes every 2 weeks than in those who used the same toothbrush for the duration of the study. Deterioration of the brushes reduced their effectiveness, but differences in gingival health status were not detected.

Manual, Ultrasonic, and Sonic Instrumentation

Q: **Are manual and ultrasonic/sonic instrumentation equally capable of improving clinical parameters?**

- A study by Drisko[29] found that the unique ability of ultrasonic/sonic scalers to use water or other chemical irrigating solutions to flush pockets during subgingival instrumentation improves reduction of pocket depth and clinical attachment gain compared with hand scaling. In addition, they noted that power-driven scalers have better access to areas that are difficult to reach, such as deep narrow defects, root grooves, and furcations. They concluded that the improvements in clinical and microbial parameters achieved by ultrasonic or sonic scalers used for periodontal debridement should equal or surpass those achieved by hand scalers.
- Nishimine and O'Leary[30] found that endotoxin values were approximately eight times greater with ultrasonic scaling compared with hand scaling.
- Cobb[1] found that as probing depth increases, the power-driven instruments become less effective because of limitations of design. When comparing the manual curette and ultrasonic instruments, the curette appears slightly more efficient but requires more effort, time, and expertise. Newly designed ultrasonic inserts appear to overcome such inherent problems.
- Leon and Vogel[31] evaluated 33 furcated molars and found that, in terms of restoring healthy gingival fluid flow and bacterial composition, in grade I furcations hand scaling and ultrasonic debridement were equally effective, but in grade II and grade III furcations ultrasonic debridement was significantly more effective than hand scaling.
- Croft et al[32] found that patients have a strong preference for ultrasonic instruments (74%).
- Dahiya et al[33] found that the greatest roughness was produced by the Gracey curette, followed by the ultrasonic tip and rotary bur. However, it took significantly longer to complete SRP procedures with the rotary bur than with the Gracey curette and ultrasonic tip.
- Several studies have reported that the use of sonic or ultrasonic instruments can result in a 20% to 50% savings in time compared with manual instrumentation when used for periodontal debridement procedures.[34]

- Lastly, Bower[35] showed that the furcation entrance is 1 mm or less 81% of the time and 0.7 mm or less 58% of the time. The ultrasonic (smaller) tip would fit better in a grade II or grade III furcation than the tip of a Gracey curette.

Q: What are the characteristics of ultrasonic and sonic scalers?

Figure 9-1 presents the characteristics of ultrasonic and sonic scalers.

Sonic	Ultrasonic	
	Magnetorestrictive	Piezoelectric
• 3,000 to 8,000 cycles/second	• 1,800 to 4,500 cycles/second	• 25,000 to 50,000 cycles/second
• Tip moves in orbital direction	• Elliptical movement of tip	• Linear movement of tip
• Increased noise	• Faster than a sonic	• Faster than a sonic
	• Example: Cavitron	

Fig 9-1 Characteristics of ultrasonic and sonic scalers.

Q: Are sonic or ultrasonic instruments more efficient?

Cobb[1] found sonic instruments to be more efficient than ultrasonic instruments, while Drisko et al[36] found similar results with ultrasonic/sonic scalers and hand instruments for removal of plaque, calculus, and endotoxin. Less damage was found at the root surfaces with the use of ultrasonic scalers at medium power compared with hand or sonic scalers. The width of ultrasonic or sonic scalers may make them a better choice than manual scalers when accessing furcations. However, measures must be taken to ensure good infection control when using power-driven scalers, which produce contaminated aerosols. There may be some clinical benefit to adding certain antimicrobials to the lavage during ultrasonic instrumentation.

Q: Do ultrasonic devices interfere with pacemakers?

Miller et al[37] found inhibition of atrial and ventricular pacing with use of an electrosurgical unit up to a distance of 10 cm, ultrasonic bath cleaner up to 30 cm, and magnetorestrictive ultrasonic scalers up to 37.5 cm. However, pacing rate and rhythm were unaffected by use of an amalgamator, electric pulp tester, composite curing light, dental handpieces, electric toothbrush, microwave oven, dental chair and light, radiography unit, and sonic scaler.

Roedig et al[38] noted interference of the ultrasonic scaler with the pacing activity of dual-chamber pacemakers (between 17 and 23 cm from the generator or leads), single-chamber pacemakers (15 cm from the generator or leads), and implantable cardioverter-defibrillators (ICDs) (7 cm from the leads). The ultrasonic cleaning system interfered with the activity of dual-chamber pacemakers (between 15 and 23 cm from the generator or leads) and single-chamber pacemakers (12 cm from the generator or leads). Pacing function was not altered by use of an electric toothbrush, electrosurgical unit, electric pulp tester, high- and low-speed handpieces, or amalgamator.

Q: Is there a difference between ultrasonic and sonic toothbrushes?

Costa et al[39] found that the use of both types of brushes resulted in significant decreases in plaque and gingival indices. However, the indices decreased more significantly in studies testing sonic brushes in orthodontic and dental implant patients. Gingival recession was not attributed to the use of the product.

Q: By how much is the blade of a Gracey curette offset?

A Gracey curette has a blade that is laterally offset by 70 degrees relative to the shank. The blade of the universal curette is situated perpendicular to the edge of the terminal shank.

Q: At what angle should the face of the curette be toward the root?

The face of the curette should be oriented at 60 degrees to the root surface.

Q: At what angle should the Gracey curette be held to the stone?

The curette should be held at an angle of 100 to 110 degrees to the stone.

Q: Is there any effect on the pulp from scaling?

Although Fischer et al[40] did not find any alteration to pulp sensitivity following scaling, dentin sensitivity to probe and/or air stimuli increased in a clinically significant manner in six patients, with five of them also experiencing sensitivity to daily stimuli. Desensitization seemed to occur naturally 2 weeks after subgingival debridement, indicating that supragingival and subgingival scaling might result in transient dentin hypersensitivity.

Reevaluation

Q: When is it an appropriate time to reevaluate a patient following SRP?

If a patient is reevaluated too soon, overtreatment may occur, but if a patient is reevaluated after too long a period, the disease might progress.

Proye et al[41] showed an initial improvement of clinical attachment at 3 weeks following SRP. No additional gain of clinical attachment occurred in the succeeding 3 months.[42] Similarly, Morrison et al[43] showed that the clinical severity of periodontitis is reduced 1 month following the "hygienic phase."

Lowenguth and Greenstein[44] concluded that prior to reevaluation following mechanical nonsurgical therapy, a minimum 3- to 4-week period should elapse, during which soft tissue healing and maturation can occur.

Maintenance

Q: Does maintenance work?

Rosling et al[45] performed a study on 50 patients, distributed into five groups, with each group receiving one of the following treatments:

- Apically repositioned flap including elimination of bony defects
- Apically repositioned flap including curettage of the bony defects, without removal of bone
- Widman flap including elimination of bony defects
- Widman flap including curettage of the bony defects, without removal of bone
- Gingivectomy including curettage of the bony defects, without removal of bone

Following treatment, oral hygiene instruction was provided, and professional dental cleanings were performed once every 2 weeks for 2 years. All surgical techniques for pocket elimination were effective in arresting periodontal disease and preventing further damage to the periodontal tissues.

Ramjford et al[46] reported that in patients who receive professional dental cleanings once every 3 months, posttreatment pocket depth and attachment levels could be maintained irrespective of personal oral hygiene (as expressed in plaque scores).

Q: What are the endpoints to successful maintenance therapy?

The endpoints to successful maintenance therapy are[47]:

- Prevent recurrence in patients who have been previously treated for gingivitis, periodontitis, and peri-implantitis
- Prevent the incidence of tooth or implant loss
- Increase the probability of locating and treating other diseases

Q: What is done during a maintenance visit?

The steps taken during a maintenance visit[48] are shown in Fig 9-2.

Fig 9-2 Workflow of a maintenance visit.

Q: What is the optimal frequency for maintenance visits?

Patients without additional attachment loss can have maintenance visits once every 6 months. However, most studies have reported that patients who have had a history of periodontal disease require maintenance visits at least four times per year.[48,49] Westfelt et al[50] found that the shorter the recall interval for maintenance visits following periodontal surgery, the better the surgical outcomes.

Q: What factors should be considered in developing an optimal maintenance schedule?

Figure 9-3 presents the factors that should be considered[51] when planning an optimal maintenance schedule.

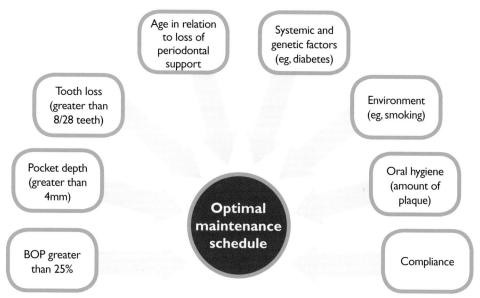

Fig 9-3 Factors to consider for an optimal maintenance schedule.

Q: What is the percentage of compliance by periodontal maintenance patients?

In a study of 961 patients, Wilson et al[52] found 16% full compliance, 49% erratic compliance, and 34% noncompliance with recommended maintenance schedules. The study found that the reasons for noncompliance included fear, lack of information, finances, and a lack of compassion from the practitioner.

In a subsequent study, Wilson et al[53] found that compliance increased from 16% in 1984 to 32% in 1991. The authors attributed this increase to factors such as efforts by office staff to increase compliance, changes in hygiene practice laws, increased public awareness of the importance of dental care, and economic considerations and concluded that compliance can be improved if the problems is recognized and addressed.

Q: What is the effect of compliance on BOP and Plaque Index?

Analysis by Miyamoto et al[54] of clinical parameters over a period of 15 years revealed that complete compliers to maintenance appointments tended to show reduction in BOP and Plaque Index compared with erratic compliers.

Q: What happens when there is a lack of supportive periodontal therapy?

In a study by Nyman et al,[55] all patients underwent presurgical treatment including case presentation and instruction in oral hygiene measures. Then patients were treated with one of the following surgical procedures:

• Apically repositioned flap including elimination of bony defects
• Apically repositioned flap including curettage of bony defects, without removal of bone
• Widman flap including elimination of bony defects
• Widman flap including curettage of bony defects, without removal of bone
• Gingivectomy including curettage of bony defects, without removal of bone

Patient assessment was performed 6, 12, and 24 months after treatment was complete. Renewed accumulation of plaque in the surgical areas resulted in recurrence of periodontal disease, including a significant further loss of attachment because the patients had poor oral hygiene and were not seen on a regular recall schedule. There was no difference in the results obtained with the various techniques; in the absence of periodontal maintenance, they were equally ineffective at preventing the recurrence of disease.

Axelsson and Lindhe[56] conducted a study on 77 patients. One-third of the patients were sent to their general dentists (GP group), and two-thirds were in a well-organized maintenance program (recalled every 2 to 3 months). Patients in the GP group had increased plaque scores and 45% loss of attachment. Patients in the maintenance program had 99% improvement and no or less than 1% attachment loss.

Q: What are some signs of disease recurrence?

Signs of disease recurrence include[57]:

• Recurrence of BOP
• Increased probing depth
• Radiographic bone loss
• Progressive mobility

Surgical and Nonsurgical Therapy

Q: **What has been shown by studies comparing surgical and nonsurgical therapy?**

Table 9-2 presents the findings of studies comparing surgical and nonsurgical therapy.

Table 9-2 | Studies comparing surgical and nonsurgical therapy

Study	Subject	Findings
Kaldahl et al[58]	Split-mouth design involving 82 patients with periodontal disease; each quadrant received one of the following: coronal scaling, root planing, modified Widman surgery, or flap with osseous resection surgery	- All the therapies reduced the pocket depth. - Osseous resection was more effective at reducing pocket depth. - Osseous resection caused the most recession. - The deeper the initial probing depth, the greater was the mean reduction of probing depth. - Root planing and modified Widman surgery produced the greatest gain of mean probing attachment in the 5- to 6-mm probing depth category.
Brayer et al[57]	Random distribution of 114 periodontally involved, single-rooted teeth designated for extraction among four operators of various experience levels for either an open or closed session of SRP	In shallow pockets, no difference was found between the two procedures; in deeper pockets (4- to 6-mm and > 6 mm), open flap SRP was more effective than closed flap SRP.
Becker et al[59]	A longitudinal study comparing scaling, osseous surgery, and modified Widman procedures	- At 5 years, there were significant decreases in gingival and plaque scores. - For the three procedures, there were significant decreases in the depth of pockets with a baseline depth of 4 to 6 mm; however, there were no differences between the methods.
Serino et al[60]	Initial outcome and long-term effect of surgical and nonsurgical treatment of advanced periodontal disease	Surgical treatment provides better short- and long-term pocket depth reduction in patients with advanced periodontal disease and may result in a reduced need for additional adjunctive therapy.

Irrigation

Q: What is the difference between supragingival and subgingival irrigation?

Supragingival irrigation is used to remove bacteria coronal to the gingival margin and reduce the chance of gingivitis. *Subgingival irrigation* is used to reduce bacteria in the pocket and prevent the initiation of periodontal disease.

Q: Should supragingival irrigation be used as monotherapy?

According to a position paper by the American Academy of Periodontology (AAP),[61] supragingival irrigation with water should not be used instead of toothbrushing.

Q: Has supragingival irrigation been shown to be effective as an adjunct in oral hygiene?

According to the AAP,[61] supragingival irrigation may not be required in patients with proficient toothbrushing skills and no gingivitis but can be of assistance in those with poor oral hygiene or gingivitis. Supragingival irrigation provides the greatest benefit to patients who do not perform adequate interproximal cleansing.

Greenstein[62] found that supragingival irrigation could enhance the oral hygiene of patients not practicing optimal plaque control but that generally no benefit beyond that provided by root planing could be achieved with subgingival irrigation.

Q: Can supragingival irrigation with antimicrobial agents be useful?

Newman et al[63] compared toothbrushing alone with adjunctive supragingival irrigation with 0.06% chlorhexidine gluconate and found the latter to significantly reduce gram-negative anaerobic rods and black-pigmented bacteroides. The effects of water irrigation on any of the assessed bacterial groups was limited.

Aziz-Gandour and Newman[64] found that low concentrations of chlorhexidine (0.02%) and metronidazole (0.05%) as irrigants in patients with periodontitis did not induce clinically significant improvements.

Q: Can irrigation induce bacteremia?

According to a position paper by the AAP,[61] irrigation does not present any particular safety hazard to systemically healthy patients given that similar levels of bacteremia were detected following activities such as toothbrushing, flossing, periodontal dressing changes, scaling, root planing, and chewing. However, when providing instructions for home irrigation to individuals requiring premedication before periodontal treatment, clinicians should be cautious because there is no specific information available regarding risk associated with home irrigation for this population.

Q: What factors are important to consider when subgingival drug delivery and irrigation are used?

The position paper by the AAP[61] indicates that the following factors should be considered when providing subgingival drug delivery and irrigation:

- Circumferential application around the teeth
- Teeth should be root planed because calculus can be an impediment
- Either a side or end port cannula can be used
- Low irrigation forces should be used (to minimize projection of bacteria to the tissues)

Q: Is subgingival irrigation effective?

The AAP position paper[61] states that although plaque indices were reduced by subgingival irrigation with medicaments, the technique did not completely eliminate inflammatory signs. When it was used alone, the number of sites with BOP was decreased. However, when it was used in conjunction with root planing, bleeding points were fewer. Most studies demonstrated a reduction in mean probing depths of less than 1 mm with subgingival irrigation. On the other hand, if irrigation was preceded by root planing, probing depths decreased 2 to 3 mm, suggesting that root planing is indicated in the achievement of probing depth reduction.

Q: How deep can supragingival and subgingival irrigation project?

The data indicate that supragingival irrigation does not routinely project solutions into deep pockets. However, subgingival irrigation via a cannula results in approximately 70% to 80% penetration of deep pockets.[61]

Pitcher et al[65] noted that solution did not routinely penetrate to the apical plaque border with mouthrinsing or direct irrigation. However, direct irrigation was partially effective, while no significant penetration of the pockets was achieved by mouthrinsing.

Q: **Is there a difference between professional and personal subgingival irrigation?**

There are no long-term studies comparing the benefit of personal versus professional administration of subgingival irrigation.

Root Conditioning

Q: **Why is root surface modification done?**

The demineralization agent removes the smear layer and facilitates new fibrous attachment and the exposure of collagen fibers to the dentin.

Q: **Is root conditioning effective?**

Chaves et al[66] used light microscopy to study the effects of SRP with and without citric acid application. They found that citric acid application did not alter the effects of SRP, and no effects to the diseased root surface were found with citric acid application as a monotherapy. Citric acid failed to penetrate the dentinal tubules and did not change the collagen content of the roots produced by SRP.

Gamal and Mailhot[67] noted that ethylenediaminetetraacetic acid (EDTA) gel conditioning for 4 minutes affords a root surface to which a maximum amount of periodontal ligament cells can adhere and propagate.

Miscellaneous

Q: **What part of the tooth experiences the most root sensitivity?**

The greatest amount of root sensitivity is experienced supragingival to the cementoenamel junction.

References

1. Cobb CM. Non-surgical pocket therapy: Mechanical. Ann Periodontol 1996;1:443–490.
2. Stambaugh RV, Dragoo M, Smith DM, Carasali L. The limits of subgingival scaling. Int J Periodontics Restorative Dent 1981;1(5):30–41.
3. Buchanan SA, Robertson PB. Calculus removal by scaling/root planing with and without surgical access. J Periodontol 1987;58:159–163.
4. Waerhaug J. Healing of the dento-epithelial junction following subgingival plaque control. II: As observed on extracted teeth. J Periodontol 1978;49:119–134.
5. Research, Science and Therapy Committee of the American Academy of Periodontology. Treatment of plaque-induced gingivitis, chronic periodontitis, and other clinical conditions. J Periodontol 2001;72:1790–1800 [erratum 2003;74:1568].

6. Loos B, Nylund K, Claffey N, Egelberg J. Clinical effects of root debridement in molar and non-molar teeth. A 2-year follow-up. J Clin Periodontol 1989;16:498–504.
7. Brayer WK, Mellonig JT, Dunlap RM, Marinak KW, Carson RE. Scaling and root planing effectiveness: The effect of root surface access and operator experience. J Periodontol 1989;60:67–72.
8. Caffesse RG, Sweeney PL, Smith BA. Scaling and root planing with and without periodontal flap surgery. J Clin Periodontol 1986;13:205–210.
9. Lindhe J, Westfelt E, Nyman S, Socransky SS, Haffajee AD. Long-term effect of surgical/nonsurgical treatment of periodontal disease. J Clin Periodontol 1984;11:448–458.
10. Goodson JM, Tanner AC, Haffajee AD, Sornberger GC, Socransky SS. Patterns of progression and regression of advanced destructive periodontal disease. J Clin Periodontol 1982;9:472–481.
11. Löe H, Anerud A, Boysen H, Morrison E. Natural history of periodontal disease in man. Rapid, moderate and no loss of attachment in Sri Lankan laborers 14 to 46 years of age. J Clin Periodontol 1986;13:431–445.
12. Lindhe J, Socransky SS, Nyman S, Haffajee A, Westfelt E. "Critical probing depths" in periodontal therapy. J Clin Periodontol 1982;9:323–336.
13. Quirynen M, De Soete M, Boschmans G, et al. Benefit of "one-stage full-mouth disinfection" is explained by disinfection and root planing within 24 hours: A randomized controlled trial. J Clin Periodontol 2006;33:639–647.
14. Greenstein G. Full-mouth therapy versus individual quadrant root planing: A critical commentary. J Periodontol 2002;73:797–812.
15. Drisko CL, Killoy WJ. Scaling and root planing: Removal of calculus and subgingival organisms. Curr Opin Dent 1991;1:74–80.
16. Coldiron NB, Yukna RA, Weir J, Caudill RF. A quantitative study of cementum removal with hand curettes. J Periodontol 1990;61:293–299.
17. Ritz L, Hefti AF, Rateitschak KH. An in vitro investigation on the loss of root substance in scaling with various instruments. J Clin Periodontol 1991;18:643–647.
18. Graves RC, Disney JA, Stamm JW. Comparative effectiveness of flossing and brushing in reducing interproximal bleeding. J Periodontol 1989;60:243–247.
19. Warren PR, Chater BV. An overview of established interdental cleaning methods. J Clin Dent 1996;7(3 special issue):65–69.
20. Bass CC. An effective method of personal oral hygiene. J LA State Med Soc 1954;106(2):57–73.
21. Carr MP, Rice GL, Horton JE. Evaluation of floss types for interproximal plaque removal. Am J Dent 2000;13:212–214.
22. Jackson MA, Kellett M, Worthington HV, Clerehugh V. Comparison of interdental cleaning methods: A randomized controlled trial. J Periodontol 2006;77:1421–1429.
23. Tu YK, Jackson M, Kellett M, Clerehugh V. Direct and indirect effects of interdental hygiene in a clinical trial. J Dent Res 2008;87:1037–1042.
24. Lang NP, Cumming BR, Löe H. Toothbrushing frequency as it relates to plaque development and gingival health. J Periodontol 1973;44:396–405.
25. Robinson PG, Deacon SA, Deery C, et al. Manual versus powered toothbrushing for oral health. Cochrane Database Syst Rev 2005;(2):CD002281.
26. Deery C, Heanue M, Deacon S, et al. The effectiveness of manual versus powered toothbrushes for dental health: A systematic review. J Dent 2004;32:197–211.
27. Rapley JW, Killoy WJ. Subgingival and interproximal plaque removal using a counter-rotational electric toothbrush and a manual toothbrush. Quintessence Int 1994;25:39–42.
28. Glaze PM, Wade AB. Toothbrush age and wear as it relates to plaque control. J Clin Periodontol 1986;13:52–56.
29. Drisko CH. Root instrumentation. Power-driven versus manual scalers, which one? Dent Clin North Am 1998;42:229–244.
30. Nishimine D, O'Leary TJ. Hand instrumentation versus ultrasonics in the removal of endotoxins from root surfaces. J Periodontol 1979;50:345–349.
31. Leon LE, Vogel RI. A comparison of the effectiveness of hand scaling and ultrasonic debridement in furcations as evaluated by differential dark-field microscopy. J Periodontol 1987;58:86–94.
32. Croft LK, Nunn ME, Crawford LC, et al. Patient preference for ultrasonic or hand instruments in periodontal maintenance. Int J Periodontics Restorative Dent 2003;23:567–573.
33. Dahiya P, Kamal R, Gupta R, Pandit N. Comparative evaluation of hand and power-driven instruments on root surface characteristics: A scanning electron microscopy study. Contemp Clin Dent 2011;2:79–83.

34. Cobb CM. Clinical significance of non-surgical periodontal therapy: An evidence-based perspective of scaling and root planing. J Clin Periodontol 2002;29(suppl 2):6–16.
35. Bower RC. Furcation morphology relative to periodontal treatment. Furcation entrance architecture. J Periodontol 1979;50:23–27.
36. Drisko CL, Cochran DL, Blieden T, et al. Position paper: Sonic and ultrasonic scalers in periodontics. Research, Science and Therapy Committee of the American Academy of Periodontology. J Periodontol 2000;71:1792–1801.
37. Miller CS, Leonelli FM, Latham E. Selective interference with pacemaker activity by electrical dental devices. Oral Surg Oral Med Oral Pathol Oral Radiol Endod 1998;85:33–36.
38. Roedig JJ, Shah J, Elayi CS, Miller CS. Interference of cardiac pacemaker and implantable cardioverter-defibrillator activity during electronic dental device use. J Am Dent Assoc 2010;141:521–526.
39. Costa MR, Marcantonio RA, Cirelli JA. Comparison of manual versus sonic and ultrasonic toothbrushes: A review. Int J Dent Hyg 2007;5:75–81.
40. Fischer C, Wennberg A, Fischer RG, Attström R. Clinical evaluation of pulp and dentine sensitivity after supragingival and subgingival scaling. Endod Dent Traumatol 1991;7:259–265.
41. Proye M, Caton J, Polson A. Initial healing of periodontal pockets after a single episode of root planing monitored by controlled probing forces. J Periodontol 1982;53:296–301.
42. Caton J, Proye M, Polson A. Maintenance of healed periodontal pockets after a single episode of root planing. J Periodontol 1982;53:420–424.
43. Morrison EC, Ramfjord SP, Hill RW. Short-term effects of initial, nonsurgical periodontal treatment (hygienic phase). J Clin Periodontol 1980;7:199–211.
44. Lowenguth RA, Greenstein G. Clinical and microbiological response to nonsurgical mechanical periodontal therapy. Periodontol 2000 1995;9:14–22.
45. Rosling B, Nyman S, Lindhe J, Jern B. The healing potential of the periodontal tissues following different techniques of periodontal surgery in plaque-free dentitions. A 2-year clinical study. J Clin Periodontol 1976;3:233–250.
46. Ramfjord SP, Morrison EC, Burgett FG, et al. Oral hygiene and maintenance of periodontal support. J Periodontol 1982;53:26–30.
47. Drisko CH. Nonsurgical periodontal therapy. Periodontol 2000 2001;25:77–88.
48. Cohen RE; Research, Science and Therapy Committee of the American Academy of Periodontology. Position paper: Periodontal maintenance. J Periodontol 2003;74:1395–401.
49. Schallhorn RG, Snider LE. Periodontal maintenance therapy. J Am Dent Assoc 1981;103:227–231.
50. Westfelt E, Nyman S, Socransky S, Lindhe J. Significance of frequency of professional tooth cleaning for healing following periodontal surgery. J Clin Periodontol 1983;10:148–156.
51. Lang NP, Brägger U, Salvi GE, Tonetti MS. Supportive periodontal therapy (SPT). In: Lindhe J, Lang NP, Karring T (eds). Clinical Periodontology and Implant Dentistry, ed 5. Oxford, UK: Blackwell Munksgaard, 2008:1303.
52. Wilson TG Jr, Glover ME, Schoen J, Baus C, Jacobs T. Compliance with maintenance therapy in a private periodontal practice. J Periodontol 1984;55:468–473.
53. Wilson TG Jr, Hale S, Temple R. The results of efforts to improve compliance with supportive periodontal treatment in a private practice. J Periodontol 1993;64:311–314.
54. Miyamoto T, Kumagai T, Jones JA, Van Dyke TE, Nunn ME. Compliance as a prognostic indicator: Retrospective study of 505 patients treated and maintained for 15 years. J Periodontol 2006;77:223–232.
55. Nyman S, Lindhe J, Rosling B. Periodontal surgery in plaque-infected dentitions. J Clin Periodontol 1977;4:240–249.
56. Axelsson P, Lindhe J. The significance of maintenance care in the treatment of periodontal disease. J Clin Periodontol 1981;8:281–294.
57. Chace R. Retreatment in periodontal practice. J Periodontol 1977;48:410–412.
58. Kaldahl WB, Kalkwarf KL, Patil KD, Dyer JK, Bates RE Jr. Evaluation of four modalities of periodontal therapy. Mean probing depth, probing attachment level and recession changes. J Periodontol 1988;59:783–793.
59. Becker W, Becker BE, Caffesse R, et al. A longitudinal study comparing scaling, osseous surgery, and modified Widman procedures: Results after 5 years. J Periodontol 2001;72:1675–1684.
60. Serino G, Rosling B, Ramberg P, Socransky SS, Lindhe J. Initial outcome and long-term effect of surgical and non-surgical treatment of advanced periodontal disease. J Clin Periodontol 2001;28:910–916.

61. Greenstein G; Research, Science and Therapy Committee of the American Academy of Periodontology. Position paper: The role of supra- and subgingival irrigation in the treatment of periodontal diseases. J Periodontol 2005;76:2015–2027.

62. Greenstein G. Nonsurgical periodontal therapy in 2000: A literature review. J Am Dent Assoc 2000;131:1580–1592.

63. Newman MG, Flemmig TF, Nachnani S, et al. Irrigation with 0.06% chlorhexidine in naturally occurring gingivitis. II. 6 months microbiological observations. J Periodontol 1990;61:427–433.

64. Aziz-Gandour IA, Newman HN. The effects of a simplified oral hygiene regime plus supragingival irrigation with chlorhexidine or metronidazole on chronic inflammatory periodontal disease. J Clin Periodontol 1986;13:228–236.

65. Pitcher GR, Newman HN, Strahan JD. Access to subgingival plaque by disclosing agents using mouthrinsing and direct irrigation. J Clin Periodontol 1980;7:300–308.

66. Chaves E, Cox C, Morrison E, Caffesse R. The effect of citric acid application on periodontally involved root surfaces. 1. An in vitro light microscopic study. Int J Periodontics Restorative Dent 1992;12:219–229.

67. Gamal AY, Mailhot JM. The effects of EDTA gel conditioning exposure time on periodontitis-affected human root surfaces: Surface topography and PDL cell adhesion. J Int Acad Periodontol 2003;5:11–22.

Surgical Therapy

Gingivectomy

Q: What are the indications for gingivectomy?

Indications for gingivectomy include[1]:

- To treat horizontal bone loss with increased pocket depth
- To reduce gingival overgrowth from medications or genetics (Fig 10-1)
- To remove soft tissue craters resulting from surgical procedures
- To improve gingival esthetics in patients with delayed passive eruption
- For crown lengthening when ostectomy is not required

Fig 10-1 Drug-induced gingival overgrowth.

Q: **What are the contraindications for a gingivectomy?**

Contraindications for gingivectomy include[2]:

- Presence of osseous defects
- Inadequate keratinized gingiva
- Base of the pocket apical to the mucogingival junction
- Inadequate vestibular depth
- Inadequate oral hygiene

Q: **Describe the gingivectomy procedure.**

The goal of gingivectomy is to eliminate gingival pockets by resection of gingival tissue. After probing the pocket to determine its base, a coronally directed external bevel incision is made using a suitable blade or knife at a 45-degree angle. The incision is made apical to the pocket but coronal to the mucogingival junction. Next the interdental incisions are made with a sharp narrow knife. After these incisions, the excised tissue should be removed with a Prichard or periosteal elevator.[1]

Osseous Surgery

Q: **What is the primary indication for periodontal flap surgery?**

The primary indication for periodontal flap surgery is to gain access to the root surface and remove bacterial deposits and calculus that may have remained following nonsurgical therapy.

Q: **What is osseous surgery? What are the indications for osseous surgery?**

First outlined by Schluger in 1949,[3] *osseous surgery* was defined as the procedures to modify bone support altered by periodontal disease either by reshaping the alveolar process to achieve physiologic form without removal of alveolar bone or by removing some alveolar bone, thus changing the position of crestal bone relative to the tooth roots.

Indications for osseous surgery, according to Schluger,[3] are:

- Failure of gingivectomy treatment
- Mesially tipped molars
- Deep isolated pockets
- Deep buccal and lingual pockets
- Saucer-shaped interproximal pockets

Q: What is the rationale for osseous surgery?

• Establish access for root debridement
• Create harmonious topology (positive architecture)
• Decrease pocket depth
• Preserve the teeth
• Allow for plaque control
• Improve prognosis
• Decrease bleeding on probing

Q: What are contraindications to osseous surgery?

• Proper follow-up and maintenance not possible
• Advanced bone loss (long-term prognosis and value of the tooth is questionable)
• Shallow pockets
• Three-wall defect (may be able to regenerate)
• Poor oral hygiene
• Medically contraindicated
• Pockets in the esthetic zone
• Poor crown-to-root ratio

Q: What can lead to failure when performing osseous surgery?

• Poor operator technique
• Failure to remove tissue tags and/or granulation tissue
• Presence of calculus
• Reverse architecture
• Improper flap placement
• Failure to remove widow's peak
• Inadequate maintenance

Q: What is osteoplasty? Ostectomy?

Both terms were first described by Friedman in 1955.[4] Friedman defined *osteoplasty* as a plastic procedure in which the periodontal pocket is eliminated and the bone reshaped to achieve physiologic contour of the bone and the gingiva overlying it. In this surgery, the bone that is reshaped is not part of the attachment apparatus, thus no bony support of the tooth or teeth is lost. Friedman defined *ostectomy* as an operative procedure in which bone that is part of the attachment apparatus is removed to eliminate a periodontal pocket and establish gingival contours that will be maintained.

Q: What determines the morphology of the defect?

- Radius of the inflammatory process
- Anatomy of the defect (thick/thin) periodontium
- Root anatomy (length and shape of the root)
- Root proximity

Different Surgical Techniques

Q: What is the difference between a full-thickness and a partial-thickness flap?

The *full-thickness flap* includes the epithelium, connective tissue, and periosteum. In a *partial-thickness flap,* the mucosa is separated from the periosteum (which is attached to the alveolar bone). The periosteal blood supply is not disturbed.

Q: Describe the modified Widman flap.

The *modified Widman flap*, first described by Ramfjord and Nissle in 1974,[5] is a flap used to provide access for root planing. Following is the procedure:

1. Initial inverse bevel incision parallel to the long axis of the teeth
2. Elevation of the mucoperiosteal flap only 2 to 3 mm from the alveolar crest
3. Crevicular incision around the neck of the teeth
4. Surgical excision of the collar of tissue around the teeth
5. Exaggerated palatal scalloping for close interproximal flap adaptation
6. Osteoplasty for flap adaptation purposes

Q: Describe the apically repositioned flap.

First described by Nabers in 1954,[6] the *apically repositioned flap* is a full-thickness reverse-beveled scalloped incision with vertical releasing incisions to the mucogingival junction. The soft tissue is displaced in an apical direction. It allows preservation of the attached gingiva following surgery.

Q: Describe the distal wedge excision.

With a *distal wedge excision,* excessive tissue distal to the last remaining tooth in the mouth can be excised to reduce the pocket. The flaps are raised, and a wedge of tissue is removed. Before suturing, the flaps are thinned.

Q: **What is an envelope flap?**

In an *envelope flap*, the horizontal incision is made at the gingival margin without any vertical incisions. The incision is used to create access.

Q: **Describe the palatal approach to osseous surgery according to Ochsenbein and Bohannan.[7]**

In 1963, Ochsenbein and Bohannan[7] described different types of defects (various interdental crater depths) and the approach that should be taken for each (Table 10-1). The majority of osteoplasty and ostectomy is done from the palatal aspect.

Table 10-1 | Palatal approach to osseous surgery

Class	Depth of the defect	Treatment
1	2 to 3 mm; thick facial and lingual tissue	10-degree palatal ramp
2 (most common)	4 to 5 mm	Facial and palatal ramp
3	6 to 7 mm	Facial and palatal ramp
4 (least common)	> 7 mm	Removal of facial and lingual tissue

Ochsenbein and Bohannan[7] advocated the palatal approach for several reasons:

• Plenty of keratinized tissue
• Increased embrasure space
• Cleansing effect of tongue
• Less resorption—greater cancellous bone
• Avoidance of exposure of the buccal furcation (maxilla root trunk is 3 mm)
• Apical slope of crest toward the palate
• Better esthetics

Q: **What were the advantages of the lingual approach to osseous surgery described by Tibbetts et al[8] in 1976?**

• The external oblique ridge is avoided.
• The furcation on the lingual is in a more apical position.
• Craters are located more lingually.
• There is better access and wider embrasure.
• The defect is located more lingually because of the lingual incline of the molars.
• The root length on the facial aspect is shorter.
• The buccal furcation is avoided (mandible root trunk is about 4 mm).
• There is greater vestibular depth on the lingual aspect.

Q: What are options for pockets found in the anterior?

- Papilla preservation flap, as described by Takei et al,[9] where a platal incision is made to allow the papilla to move in a buccal direction. However, adequate width (greater than 2 mm) of the papilla is necessary as well as a sufficient embrasure space.
- Continuous scaling and root planing.
- Perioscopy: Allows real-time indirect visualization of the root during scaling and root planing. According to Stambaugh,[10] it "can offer many patients an alternative to periodontal surgery in carefully selected sites."
- No treatment.

Q: Why are microsurgery techniques advantageous?

Cortellini and Tonetti[11] found that microsurgery can result in the following:

- Improvement of soft tissue healing
- Limited soft tissue damage
- High probability of achieving primary closure
- Limited recession
- Gains in clinical attachment level

Principles of Periodontal Surgery

Q: Why is positive architecture important when performing osseous surgery?

Positive architecture (interproximal bone coronal to the facial or lingual bone) as opposed to negative architecture (interproximal bone apical to the facial or lingual bone) allows close adaptation of the gingival tissues to the bone, which results in minimum sulcus depth.

Q: What are some general principles of periodontal surgery?

In 1977, Mörmann and Ciancio[12] outlined the following general principles of periodontal surgery:

- The flap should have a broad base to enable sufficient blood supply.
- The proportion of length to width should not exceed 2:1.
- The flap should be large enough to provide good access to the roots and bony defects.
- Partial-thickness flaps should not be too thin (to allow blood vessels to be part of the flap).

- The apical portion of periodontal flaps should be full thickness when possible.
- Partial-thickness flaps should not be used in areas of thin connective tissue because necrosis of the soft tissue may occur. This can lead to bone exposure and bone necrosis.
- There should be minimal tension during suturing.

Q: What is the average amount of supporting bone loss following osseous surgery?

Selipsky[13] found that osseous surgery results in an average of 0.6 mm of supporting bone height loss. He also found that the maximum circumferential bone loss around a tooth is 1.5 mm.

Q: Can angular defects worsen?

Papapanou and Wennström[14] found that angular defects do worsen and can be more challenging to treat if not detected early. An increased possibility of tooth loss was associated with teeth showing initial signs of angular defects.

Q: Describe how periodontal surgery is performed in your practice.

Note that there can be multiple answers to this question.

1. Scalloped incisions (when there is adequate keratinized tissue) are prepared.
2. The interproximal areas are leveled or ramped (if defect is on the lingual, ramping is performed toward the lingual) first because they will be the highest point (positive architecture). Ramping allows for less bone to be removed from the buccal aspect.
3. A round bur (#4) is used to thin the bone on the buccal and lingual aspects.
4. Physiologic architecture is developed and widow's peaks are removed using hand instruments.
5. A probe is placed interproximally to confirm that no ledges exist.
6. A continuous suture is placed.

Wound Healing

Q: What is the difference between primary, secondary, and tertiary wound healing?

- Primary: The mucosal wound edges are adjacent to one another. They are reapproximated to minimize any scarring (eg, periodontal flaps).

- Secondary: Epithelial cells must migrate (granulate in) to close the wound (eg, gingivectomy).
- Tertiary: Due to necrotic tissue or other impediment, wound closure is not possible until the impediment is removed.

Q: Describe wound healing following osseous surgery.

Table 10-2 presents results from studies of wound healing following osseous surgery.

Table 10-2 | Wound healing following osseous surgery

Study	Subject	Results
Wood et al[15]	Alveolar crest reduction following full- and partial-thickness flaps	- 0.62-mm crestal bone loss after a full-thickness flap - 0.98-mm crestal bone loss following a partial-thickness flap
Wilderman et al[16]	Histogenesis of repair following osseous surgery	- Osteoblast activity occurs 1 year after surgery - There is 1.2 mm of crestal bone loss but a gain of 0.4 mm for a net loss of 0.8 mm following surgery
Moghaddas and Stahl[17]	Alveolar bone remodeling following osseous surgery	- Mean reduction of 0.23 mm at the interradicular sites - Mean reduction of 0.55 mm at the radicular sites - Mean reduction of 0.88 mm at the furcation sites

Q: Describe healing following surgery.

Timeline for healing after surgery[18]:

- 24 hours: Blood clot connects the flap and the tooth or bone surface.
- 1 to 3 days: The space between the flap and the tooth or bone is thinner, and epithelial cells migrate to the site at a rate of 0.5 mm per day.
- 1 week: Epithelial attachment to the root occurs, and the blood clot is replaced by granulation tissue via hemidesmosomes.
- 2 weeks: Collagen fibers form parallel to the tooth surface.
- 1 month: Fully epithelialized gingival crevice.

Q: What are the patient's options when there are unresolved pocket depths?

- No treatment
- Continuous nonsurgical therapy and maintenance

- Osseous surgery for access to remove the bacteria and/or osseous reshaping for easier maintenance
- Regeneration for deeper pockets

Surgical Versus Nonsurgical Therapy

Q: **What has been shown by studies comparing surgical and nonsurgical therapy?**

See Table 9-2 in chapter 9 for a synopsis of studies comparing surgical and nonsurgical therapy.

Open Flap Curettage Versus Osseous Recontouring

Q: **Compare open flap curettage and osseous recontouring.**

In a study comparing open flap curettage and osseous recontouring, Smith et al[19] reported the following:

- Equal reduction of plaque and gingival inflammation for the two techniques
- Improved periodontal health with both techniques
- Pocket recurrence during the 6-month period following open curettage
- Maintenance of pocket reduction during the 6-month period after osseous recontouring
- Lack of bone regeneration with open curettage
- Net loss of attachment with osseous recontouring

Oral Hygiene Following Osseous Surgery

Q: **Describe the importance of oral hygiene following surgical therapy.**

In a study of 20 patients with advanced periodontal disease, Nyman et al[20] found that treatment was successful in participants in the test group, who received a professional cleaning once every 2 weeks following treatment and were able to maintain a high standard of oral hygiene. Treatment was unsuccessful in patients in the control group, who were recalled for scaling of the teeth once every 6 months and were unable to maintain good oral hygiene.

Root Resection

Q: **What are the indications for root resection?**

- Severe vertical bone loss on the root not amenable to regeneration
- Furcation invasion not maintainable
- Endodontics impossible on the root
- Vertical/horizontal root fracture

Q: **What are the contraindications for root resection?**

- Fused roots
- Advanced bone loss with unfavorable crown-to-root ratio
- Inadequate amount of root remaining on the tooth to allow it to serve as an abutment
- Remaining tooth unable to withstand normal occlusal forces
- Inadequate hygiene
- Inability to perform endodontic therapy on the remaining roots

Q: **What is the success rate of root resection?**

The most commonly resected root is the distal root of maxillary molars.

Carnevale et al[21] performed osseous recontouring and apically positioned flaps on non–furcation-involved teeth and found a 10-year survival rate of 93% for root-resected teeth and 99% at control sites.

Fuggazzotto[22] reported 96.8% and 97.0% success rates for root-resected molars and molar implants, respectively. The lowest success rate (75%) was reported for resection of the distal root of mandibular molars.

Langer et al[23] found a 62% success rate following root resection. The main reason for failure was root fracture.

ENAP

Q: **What is ENAP?**

ENAP stands for *excisional new attachment procedure*, and it was introduced by Yukna et al[24] in 1976. A knife or blade is used to perform subgingival curettage. It is an attempt to gain new attachment in suprabony pockets.

According to a position statement by the American Academy of Periodontology (AAP),[25] "Elimination of pocket epithelium by gingival curettage, ENAP or other internal bevel incision designs appears not only nearly impossible but unnecessary for long-term therapeutic goals. In addition, there are no published data that demonstrate that either curettage or ENAP are effective in periodontal regeneration. To the contrary, there is peer reviewed evidence, both in vivo and in vitro, that use of lasers for ENAP procedures and/or gingival curettage may place patients at risk for damage to root surfaces and subjacent alveolar bone that, in turn, could render these tissues incompatible to normal cell attachment and healing."

Surgical Materials

Q: What are the advantages and disadvantages of using surgical dressings?

The advantages and disadvantages of surgical dressings[26,27] are presented in Fig 10-2.

Advantages

- Protects the wound.
- Increases comfort of the patient.
- Stabilizes the flap.
- Retains the graft material.

Disadvantages

- Increases postoperative pain.
- Irritating.
- Plaque retention (increased bacteria): Powell et al[26] found that the use of a postsurgical dressing demonstrated a slightly higher rate of infection (8 infections in 300 procedures, 2.67%) than nonuse of a dressing (14 infections in 753 procedures, 1.86%).
- Jones and Cassingham[27] found that when a dressing was used, patients reported more pain and discomfort and an increased severity of pain and discomfort postoperatively. They concluded that surgical dressings were unnecessary when performing periodontal flap surgery.

Fig 10-2 Advantages and disadvantages of surgical dressings.

Q: What is Surgicel made of? Avitene?

Surgicel (Ethicon) is oxydized cellulose polymer (the unit is polyanhydro-glucuronic acid). It is used to stop postsurgical bleeding. It can be cut in different shapes and placed over the area that is bleeding.

Avitene (Davol) is microfibrillar collagen and another effective hemostatic agent. It is placed on the bleeding site with forceps.

Sutures

Q: What are the ideal properties of sutures?

The ideal properties of sutures are presented in Fig 10-3.

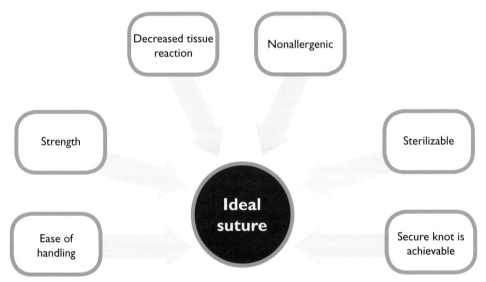

Fig 10-3 Properties of an ideal suture.

Q: What are the different types of sutures?

Figure 10-4 presents the different types of sutures.

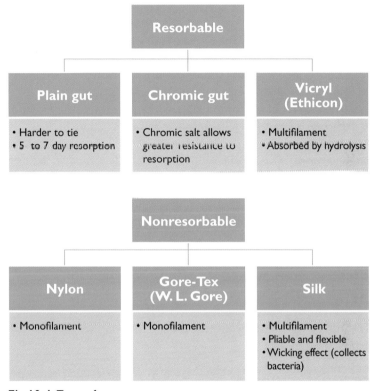

Fig 10-4 Types of sutures.

Q: What are the important principles of suturing?

Dahlberg[28] described the following principles:

- The least reactive material should be used.
- The least amount of suture material should be left beneath the flap.
- The suture should be placed close to the tissue.
- The suture should be removed as soon as possible.

Q: Describe the different techniques for suturing.

- Interrupted: Used when the facial and lingual aspects require similar tension and heights. It is a good choice for a replaced or coronally repositioned flap.
- Sling: The position of the facial or lingual flap is independent of the opposing flap.
- Mattress: Allows for eversion of the edges of the wound and maximum tissue coverage; the vertical mattress suture avoids suture material under the flap, while the horizontal mattress suture can prevent clot destabilization.
- Periosteal: Used to apically displace partial-thickness flaps.
- Figure 8 suture: Helpful in extraction sites when primary closure cannot always be achieved. It looks like a horizontal number 8.

Newell and Brunsvold[29] explained that long, thin papillae should be sutured with a vertical mattress suture, while short, wide papillae should be sutured with a horizontal mattress suture.

Postoperative Period

Q: What instructions should a patient be given following surgery?

Following are instructions to provide to patients following surgery (Sims T, personal communication, 2012):

- Care of your mouth: Immediately after surgery, keep ice-cold water or other cold foods, such as ice cream or frozen yogurt, in your mouth for 6 to 8 hours. Do not brush your teeth in the areas that have dressing or sutures. Perform normal cleaning of all teeth that did not undergo surgery.
- Activity: Reduce your activity following surgery. No running, weightlifting, or any strenuous aerobic activity or contact sports for 48 hours.
- Discomfort: Following all types of surgery, you can expect some discomfort. Take your pain medication as prescribed. Do not drink alcoholic beverages in combination with pain medication.
- Swelling: In some cases swelling may be expected, but it will go away in 3 to 4 days.
- Eating: Eat only cold, soft foods on the day of surgery. After the first day, stay on a soft but balanced diet. Do not eat hard, crunchy, or spicy foods.
- Smoking: Do not smoke following surgery. Tobacco smoke is an irritant and delays healing of the tissue. Refrain from smoking for as long as possible.

Miscellaneous

Q: What is the postinfection rate following periodontal surgery?

In a retrospective study of 395 patients that included 1,053 fully documented surgical procedures, Powell et al[26] reviewed surgical techniques such as osseous resective surgery, flap curettage, distal wedge procedures, gingivectomy, root resection, guided tissue regeneration, dental implant surgery, epithelialized free soft tissue autografts, subepithelial connective tissue autografts, coronally positioned flaps, sinus augmentations, and ridge preservation or augmentation procedures. Infection, defined as increasing and progressive swelling with the presence of suppuration, was found at a rate of 2.09% (22/1,053).

Pack and Haber[30] discovered 6/268 (2.2%) surgeries with infection when osseous surgery was performed, whereas 2/336 (0.6%) infections were noted with periodontal surgery without osteoplasty or ostectomy.

Q: How much blood loss occurs in periodontal surgery?

In a study of 26 patients requiring open flap debridement or regeneration, Zigdon et al[31] reported intraoperative blood loss ranging from 6.0 to 145.1 mL, with an overall mean of 59.47 ± 38.2 mL. The volume of blood loss was not related to the amount of local anesthetic, the size of the surgical field, or the duration of the surgery. They concluded that a minimal amount of blood is lost during periodontal surgery.

Baab et al[32] found that mandibular periodontal surgery caused greater blood loss than maxillary surgery (about a 40-mL difference).

References

1. Rose LF, Mealey BL, Genco RJ, Cohen DW. Periodontics: Medicine, Surgery, and Implants. St Louis: Elsevier Mosby, 2004:505–506.
2. Serio FG, Hawley C. Manual of Clinical Periodontics. Hudson, OH: Lexi-Comp, 2002.
3. Schluger S. Osseous resection: A basic principle in periodontal surgery. Oral Surg Oral Med Oral Pathol 1949;2:316–325.
4. Friedman N. Periodontal osseous surgery: Osteoplasty and osteoectomy. J Periodontol 1955;26:269.
5. Ramfjord SP, Nissle RR. The modified Widman flap. J Periodontol 1974;45:601–607.
6. Nabers CL. Repositioning the attached gingiva. J Periodontol 1954;25:38–39.
7. Ochsenbein C, Bohannan HM. The palatal approach to osseous surgery. I. Rationale. J Periodontol 1963;34:60.
8. Tibbetts LS Jr, Ochsenbein C, Loughlin DM. Rationale for the lingual approach to mandibular osseous surgery. Dent Clin North Am 1976;20:61–78.
9. Takei HH, Han TJ, Carranza FA Jr, Kenney EB, Lekovic V. Flap technique for periodontal bone implants. Papilla preservation technique. J Periodontol 1985;56:204–210.
10. Stambaugh RV. A clinician's 3-year experience with perioscopy. Compend Contin Educ Dent 2002;23:1061–1070.

11. Cortellini P, Tonetti MS. Microsurgical approach to periodontal regeneration. Initial evaluation in a case cohort. J Periodontol 2001;72:559 569.

12. Mörmann W, Ciancio SG. Blood supply of human gingiva following periodontal surgery. A fluorescein angiographic study. J Periodontol 1977;48:681–692.

13. Selipsky H. Osseous surgery—How much need we compromise? Dent Clin North Am 1976;20:79–106.

14. Papapanou PN, Wennström JL. The angular bony defect as indicator of further alveolar bone loss. J Clin Periodontol 1991;18:317–322.

15. Wood DL, Hoag PM, Donnenfeld OW, Rosenfeld LD. Alveolar crest reduction following full and partial thickness flaps. J Periodontol 1972;43:141–144.

16. Wilderman MN, Pennel BM, King K, Barron JM. Histogenesis of repair following osseous surgery. J Periodontol 1970;41:551–565.

17. Moghaddas H, Stahl SS. Alveolar bone remodeling following osseous surgery. A clinical study. J Periodontol 1980;51:376–381.

18. Newman MG, Takei H, Klokkevold PR, Carranza FA. Carranza's Clinical Periodontology, ed 11. St Louis: Elsevier Saunders, 2012:935.

19. Smith DH, Ammons WF Jr, Van Belle G. A longitudinal study of peridontal status comparing osseous recontouring with flap curettage. I. Results after 6 months. J Periodontol 1980;51:367–375.

20. Nyman S, Rosling B, Lindhe J. Effect of professional tooth cleaning on healing after periodontal surgery. J Clin Periodontol 1975;2:80–86.

21. Carnevale G, Pontoriero R, di Febo G. Long-term effects of root-resective therapy in furcation-involved molars. A 10-year longitudinal study. J Clin Periodontol 1998;25:209–214.

22. Fugazzotto PA. A comparison of the success of root resected molars and molar position implants in function in a private practice: Results of up to 15-plus years. J Periodontol 2001;72:1113–1123.

23. Langer B, Stein SD, Wagenberg B. An evaluation of root resections. A ten-year study. J Periodontol 1981;52:719–722.

24. Yukna RA, Bowers GM, Lawrence JJ, Fedi PF Jr. A clinical study of healing in humans following the excisional new attachment procedure. J Periodontol 1976;47:696–700.

25. American Academy of Periodontology. Statement Regarding Use of Dental Lasers for Excisional New Attachment Procedure (ENAP). http://www.perio.org/resources-products/enap_laser.htm. Accessed 28 September 2012.

26. Powell CA, Mealey BL, Deas DE, McDonnell HT, Moritz AJ. Post-surgical infections: Prevalence associated with various periodontal surgical procedures. J Periodontol 2005;76:329–333.

27. Jones TM, Cassingham RJ. Comparison of healing following periodontal surgery with and without dressings in humans. J Periodontol 1979;50:387–393.

28. Dahlberg WH. Incisions and suturing: Some basic considerations about each in periodontal flap surgery. Dent Clin North Am 1969;13:149–159.

29. Newell DH, Brunsvold MA. A modification of the "curtain technique" incorporating an internal mattress suture. J Periodontol 1985;56:484–487.

30. Pack PD, Haber J. The incidence of clinical infection after periodontal surgery. A retrospective study. J Periodontol 1983;54:441–443.

31. Zigdon H, Levin L, Filatov M, Oettinger-Barak O, Machtei EE. Intraoperative bleeding during open flap debridement and regenerative periodontal surgery. J Periodontol 2012;83:55–60.

32. Baab DA, Ammons WF Jr, Selipsky H. Blood loss during periodontal flap surgery. J Periodontol 1977;48:693–698.

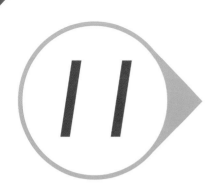

Mucogingival Therapy

Background

Q: What is the definition of mucogingival therapy?

A 1996 consensus report by the American Academy of Periodontology defines *mucogingival therapy* as "non-surgical and surgical correction of the defects in morphology, position and/or amount of soft tissue and underlying bone."[1]

In 1988, Miller[2] coined the term *periodontal plastic surgery* to include not only treatment of recession and problems associated with attached gingiva but also "correction of ridge form, exposing unerupted teeth for orthodontic treatment, crown lengthening for esthetic purposes, and frenal surgery."

Q: What is the prevalence of dehiscence and fenestration in the maxilla and the mandible?

Table 11-1 presents the prevalence of dehiscence and fenestration.[3]

Table 11-1	Prevalence of dehiscence and fenestration	
	Maxilla	Mandible
Dehiscence (%)	6	14
Fenestration (%)	17	6

Q: What are the endpoints of success with mucogingival therapy?

- Gingival augmentation
- Prevention or cessation of recession
- Facilitation of plaque control
- Elimination of an aberrant frenum
- Increased vestibular depth
- Decreased root sensitivity
- Decreased inflammation

Q: What are some side effects from mucogingival therapy?

- Increased bleeding
- Bone exposure
- Color discrepancies
- Necrosis of donor site
- Herpetic lesions
- Delayed healing

Gingival Recession

Q: What causes gingival recession?

- Abrasive and traumatic toothbrushing habits
- Periodontal inflammation
- Tooth positioned too buccal
- Frenal and muscle attachment encroachment
- Orthodontic movement
- Underlying bony dehiscence
- Genetics
- Invasion of biologic width

Q: What are the consequences of gingival recession?

Figure 11-1 presents the consequences of gingival recession.[4]

Pain from the exposed dentin

Poor esthetics

Inflammation and plaque retention

Root caries and tooth abrasion

Fig 11-1 Consequences of gingival recession.

Q: **What is the prevalence of gingival recession?**

According to a study by Albandar and Kingman,[5] the prevalence of ≥ 1 mm recession is 58% in individuals 30 years and older and increases with age. The prevalence of recession is 37.8% in those aged 30 to 39 years and increases to 90.4% in persons aged 80 to 90 years.

Q: **Once recession is present, can it worsen?**

Serino et al[6] found a 3-mm recession site worsened 67% of the time. A 4-mm recession site worsened 98% of the time.

Q: **Is there a minimum amount of attached gingiva required to avoid recession?**

Studies by Lang and Loe[7]: A minimum of 2 mm of keratinized gingiva (1 mm attached and 1 mm free gingiva) is needed to maintain gingival health.

Studies by Maynard and Wilson[8]: If there is good oral hygiene, a lack of attached gingiva does not result in recession.

Q: **How much attached gingiva is required around restorations?**

According to studies by Maynard and Wilson,[8] 5 mm of keratinized attached gingiva composed of 2 mm of free gingiva and 3 mm of attached gingiva is needed to meet restorative goals.

Q: **How does widening the attached gingiva help the patient?**

- Enhances plaque control around the gingival margin
- Improves esthetics
- Reduces inflammation around the restored teeth

Classification of Recession

Q: **What is Miller's classification[9] of soft tissue recession?**

Miller's classification[9] of soft tissue recession is shown in Fig 11-2.

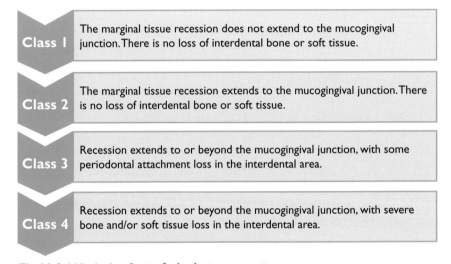

Class 1	The marginal tissue recession does not extend to the mucogingival junction. There is no loss of interdental bone or soft tissue.
Class 2	The marginal tissue recession extends to the mucogingival junction. There is no loss of interdental bone or soft tissue.
Class 3	Recession extends to or beyond the mucogingival junction, with some periodontal attachment loss in the interdental area.
Class 4	Recession extends to or beyond the mucogingival junction, with severe bone and/or soft tissue loss in the interdental area.

Fig 11-2 Miller's classification[9] of soft tissue recession.

Q: **What is the expected root coverage for each of Miller's classes?**

- Class 1: 100% root coverage.
- Class 2: 100% root coverage.
- Class 3: Partial root coverage is anticipated 50% to 70% of the time.
- Class 4: Root coverage is not anticipated; the success rate is less than 10%.

Q: **Describe the Sullivan and Atkins classification**[10] **of mucogingival defects.**

Figure 11-3 presents the Sullivan and Atkins classification[10] of mucogingival defects.

Deep-wide	Shallow-wide	Deep-narrow	Shallow-narrow
The deep-wide defect is the most difficult area to treat. The graft should cover at least 5 mm of the connective tissue bed. Expect 1 to 2 mm of coverage.	Expect 1 to 2 mm of new tissue over the apical portion.	Rarely seen; expect complete coverage.	Maintain by conservative therapy.

Fig 11-3 Sullivan and Atkins classification.[10]

Q: **How are alveolar ridge defects classified?**

Alveolar ridge defects are classified by the Seibert[11] classification:

- Class 1: Buccopalatal loss of tissue with normal apicocoronal ridge height
- Class 2: Apicocoronal loss of tissue with normal buccopalatal ridge width
- Class 3: Combination defect—loss of both width and height of the ridge

Technique

Q: **What is the technique for placement of a free gingival graft versus a connective tissue graft?**

The techniques for placement of free gingival grafts and connective tissue (CT) grafts are presented in Fig 11-4.

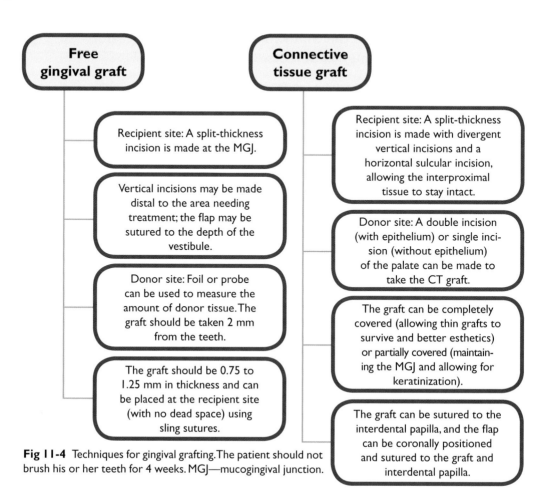

Free gingival graft

Recipient site: A split-thickness incision is made at the MGJ.

Vertical incisions may be made distal to the area needing treatment; the flap may be sutured to the depth of the vestibule.

Donor site: Foil or probe can be used to measure the amount of donor tissue. The graft should be taken 2 mm from the teeth.

The graft should be 0.75 to 1.25 mm in thickness and can be placed at the recipient site (with no dead space) using sling sutures.

Connective tissue graft

Recipient site: A split-thickness incision is made with divergent vertical incisions and a horizontal sulcular incision, allowing the interproximal tissue to stay intact.

Donor site: A double incision (with epithelium) or single incision (without epithelium) of the palate can be made to take the CT graft.

The graft can be completely covered (allowing thin grafts to survive and better esthetics) or partially covered (maintaining the MGJ and allowing for keratinization).

The graft can be sutured to the interdental papilla, and the flap can be coronally positioned and sutured to the graft and interdental papilla.

Fig 11-4 Techniques for gingival grafting. The patient should not brush his or her teeth for 4 weeks. MGJ—mucogingival junction.

Q: **What are the advantages of a CT graft compared with a free gingival graft?**

- Palate can heal by primary intention.
- Patient has less pain.
- CT graft is more esthetic (better color match).

Q: **Does the orientation of the CT graft affect root coverage or gingival augmentation?**

Al-Zahrani et al[12] studied 16 pairs of bilateral gingival recessions (Miller Class 1 and Class 2). For each patient (13 patients), one side received a CT graft with the superficial surface toward the gingival flap, and the other side had the same surface toward the root surface. The study measured Plaque Index, Gingival Index, probing depth, gingival recession, root coverage, and relative clinical attachment level. The study found that neither root coverage nor gingival augmentation were significantly altered by the surface orientation of a CT graft.

Lafzi et al[13] had a similar finding. Their study found that the short-term clinical outcome of a CT graft with a coronally advanced flap is not affected by orientation of the CT graft.

Q: **Are there different outcomes when placing grafts using a microsurgery versus a macrosurgery technique?**

Burkhardt and Lang[14] found greater vascularization and root coverage immediately, 3 days, and 7 days following microsurgery compared with outcomes at the same time points when the macrosurgery technique was used.

Wound Healing

Q: **Describe the wound healing of a free gingival graft.**

Following is the timeline for wound healing of a free gingival graft according to Gargiulo and Arrocha[15]:

- 0 to 2 days: Plasmatic circulation
- 2 to 4 days: Vascular invasion
- 4 to 7 days: Connective tissue attachment
- 10 days: Bridge of vascular channels
- 21 days: Connective tissue is well organized

Q: **How much shrinkage can occur after placing the graft?**

At 360 days after grafting, Mormann et al[16] found the percentages of shrinkage to be 45% very thin, 44% thin, and 38% intermediate. Most shrinkage occurs within the first 6 weeks.

Q: **How much creeping attachment can be expected?**

According to Matter,[17] 0.89 mm of creeping attachment is expected.

Anatomy for Mucogingival Therapy

Q: **When harvesting a CT graft, which area has the greatest soft tissue thickness?**

The tuberosity at the mid-distal position has the greatest soft tissue thickness.

Q: **What is the average distance from the greater palatine foramen to the cementoenamel junction (CEJ)?**

Following are the average distances from the greater palatine foramen to the CEJ based on the depth of the palate. According to Reiser et al,[18] these figures are important to consider when taking donor tissue from the palate.

- Deep palate: 17 mm
- Average depth palate: 12 mm
- Shallow palate: 7 mm

Q: **Is it more effective to place a graft on bone or on periosteum?**

- Bone: James and McFall[19] believed that there could be 1.5 to 2 times more shrinkage if a graft were placed on periosteum instead of bone. Matter and Cimasoni[20] found that grafts placed on denuded bone shrank 25% and grafts placed on periosteum shrank 50%.
- Periosteum: Caffesse and Guinard[21] believed that there is delayed remodeling of grafts placed on bone. Lindhe et al[22] observed greater bone resorption on bone than on periosteum.

Different Flap Techniques

Q: **Describe the laterally positioned flap.**

Grupe and Warren[23] described the technique in which a split-thickness incision is made one papilla distal or mesial to the affected site beyond the mucogingival junction. The flap is allowed to slide over to the adjacent recipient site. The flap should be made wider than the recipient site. A pedicle flap should have an adequate zone of keratinized tissue in terms of thickness and quantity adjacent to the area of recession. The patient should have an adequate vestibule as well.

Q: **Describe the double papilla flap.**

The double papilla pedicle flap was first introduced by Cohen and Ross[24] in 1968. According to Cohen and Ross, the procedure is useful for treating recession occurring on the lingual or facial gingiva, and it avoids the need for destruction of the interdental papillae on either side of the area of denudation. The papilla from each tooth is moved over the facial or lingual aspect of the recipient tooth. This technique allows for a dual blood supply. A sling suture is used at the end of the procedure.

Q: Describe the semilunar technique.

Tarnow[25] described a technique that allows the practitioner to make a split-thickness incision parallel to the outline of the gingival margin and 2 mm away from the papilla. This technique is reserved for limited recession. Sutures are not needed for this technique.

Q: When should a coronally positioned flap be used?

The coronally positioned flap was first described by Bernimoulin in 1981.[26] A split-thickness incision is made with vertical incisions that go beyond the mucogingival junction. Some guidelines to perform a coronally positioned flap include:

- Minimum tissue thickness of 0.8 mm (Baldi et al[27])
- Shallow recession of less than 4 mm
- Miller class I
- Keratinized attached tissue greater than 3 mm
- There should be minimal to no flap tension
- The flap should be placed 2.5 mm coronal to the CEJ

Zucchelli et al[28] found that a coronally positioned flap without vertical incisions (ie, envelope flap) had an increased chance of complete root coverage and decreased postoperative morbidity.

Alloderm

Q: Describe alloderm and the technique used to place it.

Alloderm is human dermis made of a matrix of collagen, elastin, vascular channels, and protein that support its revascularization. It has been processed to remove the epidermis and cells that can lead to tissue rejection and graft rejection without damaging the matrix. Alloderm can be placed in a tunnel as described below:

1. Hydrate the alloderm.
2. Scale and root plane the teeth in the affected site.
3. Prepare the site 3 mm apical to the papilla tip and leave one papilla intact.
4. Place alloderm and suture for stability.
5. Place sling sutures (polypropylene sutures are recommended).

Q: What is the main contraindication to alloderm?

Do not use alloderm if the patient is allergic to gentomycin.

Q: Is an autogenous graft or alloderm more effective?

According to studies by Wei et al,[29] alloderm is less effective in increasing attached keratinized tissue and can lead to more shrinkage. However, the study found better esthetics with alloderm. Henderson et al[30] found that with alloderm, there was no creeping attachment and a gain of keratinized attachment of about 1 mm.

A meta-analysis by Gapski et al[31] noted no statistically significant dissimilarities between surgeries using alloderm and other mucogingival surgeries.

Guided Tissue Regeneration (GTR)

Q: Why would it be beneficial to use GTR as opposed to a soft tissue procedure alone?

- There is not a second surgical site.
- Bone may regenerate.

A challenge is that it is difficult to create enough space for generating tissue between the root surface and membrane.

In a 10-year study comparing CT grafts with GTR, Nickles et al[32] found that CT grafts had a better treatment outcome but caused greater postoperative discomfort compared with GTR.

Q: Is the thickness of the flap a predictor of root coverage?

Table 11-2 presents the percentage of root coverage based on the thickness of the flap according to Harris.[33]

Table 11-2 | Thickness of the flap and percentage of root coverage

Technique	Thin flap (%)	Thick flap (%)
CT with a double pedicle flap	100	95.9
Membrane placement	26.7	96

Q: **Based on periodontal informational papers,[34] what is the mean defect coverage for the free gingival graft, pedicle graft, CT graft, coronally positioned graft, GTR, and alloderm?**

Table 11-3 presents the mean defect coverage for different grafting techniques and alloderm.

Table 11-3 | Mean defect coverage using different techniques

Free gingival graft	Pedicle graft	CT graft	Coronally positioned graft	GTR (Resorbable membrane)	GTR (Non-resorbable membrane)	Alloderm
69%	67%	84%	78%	72%	73%	86%

Enamel Matrix Derivative (EMD)

Q: **Has EMD (porcine amelogenin) shown any improvement in mucogingival therapy?**

EMD (eg, Emdogain, Straumann) placed with a coronally placed flap or CT graft seems to accelerate soft tissue healing. According to a position paper,[34] the addition of Emdogain to a flap had a mean defect coverage of 86%.

Frenectomy

Q: **Is there a need for frenectomy?**

According to Ward,[35] a frenectomy and free gingival graft increases the attached gingiva and decreases recession.

According to a study of 1,000 children by Addy et al,[36] frenal attachment had a minor influence on plaque and gingivitis and did not justify mucogingival therapy.

Q: Is there a relationship between orthodontics and recession?

According to Bollen et al,[37] there is a relationship between orthodontics and recession. The study found 0.03 mm of recession.

Loss of the Papilla

Q: What causes loss of the papilla?

- Loss of periodontal support
- Trauma
- Abnormal tooth shape

Q: What is the classification of loss of papilla height by Nordland and Tarnow?[38]

Following is the classification of loss of papilla height by Nordland and Tarnow[38]:

- Normal: Fills the embrasure space
- Class 1: Tip of the papilla is between the interproximal contact and interproximal CEJ
- Class 2: Tip of the papilla is between the interproximal CEJ and the facial CEJ
- Class 3: Tip of the papilla is apical to the facial CEJ

Q: What occurs when papillae are lost?

- Phonetic problems
- Interproximal food entrapment
- Esthetic impairment

Q: Is it possible for the papillae to be reconstructed?

The success may depend on the distance between the bone crest and the interproximal contact point, as reported by Tarnow et al.[39] According to many studies, predictable reconstruction of lost interproximal papillae is not yet possible.

Gingival Overgrowth and Excessive Gingival Display

Q: **What can cause gingival overgrowth?**

The following may cause gingival overgrowth[4]:

- Plaque
- Hormones (pregnancy, contraceptives)
- Hereditary gingival fibromatosis
- Scurvy
- Drugs
- Mouth breathing
- Neoplasia
- Granulomatous conditions

Q: **What is excessive gingival display and why does it occur?**

Excessive gingival display is a condition in which a significant amount of gingiva is visible when the patient smiles. It may be caused by:

- Failure of the gingiva to migrate apically after eruption of the teeth
- Vertical maxillary excess
- Upper lip incompetence

Q: **What is Coslet et al's classification[40] of altered passive eruption? What treatment is recommended for each?**

Figure 11-5 presents the classification of altered passive eruption by Coslet et al[40] and the associated treatment approaches.

Type 1: The gingival margin is incisal or occlusal to the CEJ, and the MGJ is apical to the crest of bone

Type 2: The gingival dimension is normal. The free gingival margin is incisal or occlusal to the CEJ, and the MGJ is positioned at the CEJ.

Subtype A: Alveolar crest is 1.5 to 2 mm apical to the CEJ

Treatment: Gingivectomy

Subtype A: Alveolar crest is 1.5 to 2 mm apical to the CEJ

Treatment: Apically positioned flap without osseous resection

Subtype B: Alveolar crest is coincident with the CEJ

Treatment: Gingivectomy or scalloped inverse bevel

Subtype B: Alveolar crest is coincident with the CEJ

Treatment: Apically positioned flap with osseous resection

Fig 11-5 Coslet et al classification[40] of altered passive eruption. MGJ—mucogingival junction.

Crown Lengthening

Q: What are the indications for crown lengthening?

- Subgingival fracture/caries
- Endodontic pin/post perforation
- Root resorption
- Inadequate height available for the restoration (Fig 11-6)
- Esthetically short crown
- Altered passive eruption
- Biologic width would be violated during a restorative procedure

Fig 11-6 (a) Before crown lengthening. (b) After crown lengthening.

Q: **What are some important considerations when deciding to remove soft tissue or bone during a crown lengthening procedure?**

If there is greater than 3 mm of soft tissue between the bone and gingival margin with adequate attached gingiva, crown lengthening by gingivectomy is possible. However, if there is less than 3 mm of soft tissue between the bone and the gingival margin or less than adequate attached gingiva, osseous recontouring is needed.

Q: **What are some essential technical factors to consider when performing crown lengthening?**

- A full-thickness mucoperiosteal flap should be made.
- A minimum ferrule of 1.5 mm should be allowed for retention.
- A 6-degree taper and a minimum of 3.5 mm (1.5 mm of ferrule and about 2 mm of biologic width) of circumferential tooth structure are required. However, Wagenberg et al[41] noted that 5 to 5.25 mm of tooth structure above the osseous crest is necessary.
- In the case of caries/fracture, at least 1 mm of sound tooth structure should be provided above the gingival margin for proper restoration.
- Esthetics and the final position of the incisal edge (anterior cases): The average width-to-length ratio of a maxillary central incisor is 75% to 80%.
- The flap should be apically positioned to the new level of the alveolar crest. Deas et al[42] found that the position of the flap in relation to the alveolar crest at suturing seems to be related to tissue rebound. The closer the tissue is sutured to the alveolar crest, the greater the chance of tissue rebound.
- At least 8 weeks should be allowed following surgery before restorative procedures are performed. Brägger et al[43] found 2 to 4 mm of recession of the gingival margin between 6 weeks and 6 months postoperatively in 12% of crown lengthening procedures.

Restorative Considerations

Q: **Is it possible to obtain root coverage over caries lesions?**

According to Goldstein et al,[44] carious root coverage (92%) is as predictable as coverage of intact roots (97%).

Q: **How much tissue healing needs to occur before restorative treatment can be initiated?**

Two months of tissue healing is required before restorative treatment is initiated.

Q: **Which restorative pontic is ideal for gingival tissues?**

An ovate pontic is ideal because it tapers to the level of tissue on the palate to allow for hygiene access. It also mimics the natural tooth contour and allows for an esthetic outcome.[45] Spear[46] advocated an ovate pontic because it adapts to the site with a flat or concave outline. However, most restorative dentists prescribe a modified ridge lap because it has better esthetics in areas of reduced bone.

Miscellaneous

Q: **What are the indications for soft tissue versus hard tissue grafting?**

Soft tissue grafting
- Mild to moderate defects
- Horizontal defects
- Available tissue

Hard tissue grafting
- Moderate to severe defects (greater than 4 mm)
- Horizontal and vertical defects
- Inadequate soft tissue quality

Q: **What procedures require a vestibule to be successful?**

CT grafts, pedicle grafts, and tunnel techniques require the presence of a vestibule.

Q: **Is it possible to obtain molar root coverage?**

According to a study of 50 cases by Harris,[47] it is possible to achieve 91.1% molar root coverage.

References

1. Prato GP. Advances in mucogingival surgery. J Int Acad Periodontol 2000;2:24–27.
2. Miller PD Jr. Regenerative and reconstructive periodontal plastic surgery. Mucogingival surgery. Dent Clin North Am 1988;32:287–306.
3. Elliott JR, Bowers GM. Alveolar dehiscence and fenestration. Periodontics 1963;1:245–248.
4. Clerehugh V, Tugnait A, Genco RJ. Periodontology at a Glance. Oxford: Wiley-Blackwell, 2009: 64,66.
5. Albandar JM, Kingman A. Gingival recession, gingival bleeding, and dental calculus in adults 30 years of age and older in the United States, 1988-1994. J Periodontol 1999;70:30–43.
6. Serino G, Wennström JL, Lindhe J, Eneroth L. The prevalence and distribution of gingival recession in subjects with a high standard of oral hygiene. J Clin Periodontol 1994;21:57–63.
7. Lang NP, Löe H. The relationship between the width of keratinized gingiva and gingival health. J Periodontol 1972;43:623–627.
8. Maynard JG Jr, Wilson RD. Physiologic dimensions of the periodontium significant to the restorative dentist. J Periodontol 1979;50:170–174.
9. Miller PD Jr. A classification of marginal tissue recession. Int J Periodontics Restorative Dent 1985;5(2):8–13.
10. Sullivan HC, Atkins JH. Free autogenous gingival grafts. I. Principles of successful grafting. Periodontics 1968;6:121–129.
11. Seibert JS. Reconstruction of deformed, partially edentulous ridges, using full thickness onlay grafts. Part I. Technique and wound healing. Compend Contin Educ Dent 1983;4:437–453.
12. Al-Zahrani MS, Bissada NF, Ficara AJ, Cole B. Effect of connective tissue graft orientation on root coverage and gingival augmentation. Int J Periodontics Restorative Dent 2004;24:65–69.
13. Lafzi A, Mostofi Zadeh Farahani R, Abolfazli N, Amid R, Safaiyan A. Effect of connective tissue graft orientation on the root coverage outcomes of coronally advanced flap. Clin Oral Investig 2007;11:401–408.
14. Burkhardt R, Lang NP. Coverage of localized gingival recessions: Comparison of micro- and macrosurgical techniques. J Clin Periodontol 2005;32:287–293.
15. Gargiulo AW, Arrocha R. Histo-clinical evaluation of free gingival grafts. Periodontics 1967;5:285–291.
16. Mörmann W, Schaer F, Firestone AR. The relationship between success of free gingival grafts and transplant thickness. Revascularization and shrinkage—A one year clinical study. J Periodontol 1981;52:74–80.
17. Matter J. Creeping attachment of free gingival grafts. A five-year follow-up study. J Periodontol 1980;51:681–685.
18. Reiser GM, Bruno JF, Mahan PE, Larkin LH. The subepithelial connective tissue graft palatal donor site: Anatomic considerations for surgeons. Int J Periodontics Restorative Dent 1996;16:130–137.
19. James WC, McFall WT Jr. Placement of free gingival grafts on denuded alveolar bone. Part I: Clinical evaluations. J Periodontol 1978;49:283–290.
20. Matter J, Cimasoni G. Creeping attachment after free gingival grafts. J Periodontol 1976;47:574–579.
21. Caffesse RG, Guinard EA. Treatment of localized gingival recessions. Part II. Coronally repositioned flap with a free gingival graft. J Periodontol 1978;49:357–361.
22. Lindhe J, Nyman S, Karring T. Connective tissue reattachment as related to presence or absence of alveolar bone. J Clin Periodontol 1984;11:33–40.
23. Grupe HE, Warren RF. Repair of gingival defects by a sliding flap operation. J Periodontol 1956;27:92–95.
24. Cohen DW, Ross SE. The double papillae repositioned flap in periodontal therapy. J Periodontol 1968;39:65–70.
25. Tarnow DP. Semilunar coronally repositioned flap. J Clin Periodontol 1986;13:182–185.
26. Bernimoulin JP. Use of a free mucous membrane transplant in mucogingival surgery with special consideration for the treatment of recession [in German]. ZWR 1981;90(12):52–55.
27. Baldi C, Pini-Prato G, Pagliaro U, et al. Coronally advanced flap procedure for root coverage. Is flap thickness a relevant predictor to achieve root coverage? A 19-case series. J Periodontol 1999;70:1077–1084.

28. Zucchelli G, Mele M, Mazzotti C, Marzadori M, Montebugnoli L, De Sanctis M. Coronally advanced flap with and without vertical releasing incisions for the treatment of multiple gingival recessions: A comparative controlled randomized clinical trial. J Periodontol 2009;80:1083–1094.

29. Wei PC, Laurell L, Geivelis M, Lingen MW, Maddalozzo D. Acellular dermal matrix allografts to achieve increased attached gingiva. Part 1. A clinical study. J Periodontol 2000;71:1297–1305.

30. Henderson RD, Drisko CH, Greenwell H. Root coverage using Alloderm acellular dermal graft material. J Contemp Dent Pract 1999;1:24–30.

31. Gapski R, Parks CA, Wang HL. Acellular dermal matrix for mucogingival surgery: A meta-analysis. J Periodontol 2005;76:1814–1822.

32. Nickles K, Ratka-Krüger P, Neukranz E, Raetzke P, Eickholz P. Ten-year results after connective tissue grafts and guided tissue regeneration for root coverage. J Periodontol 2010;81:827–836.

33. Harris RJ. A comparative study of root coverage obtained with guided tissue regeneration utilizing a bioabsorbable membrane versus the connective tissue with partial-thickness double pedicle graft. J Periodontol 1997;68:779–790.

34. Greenwell H, Fiorellini J, Giannobile W, et al. Oral reconstructive and corrective considerations in periodontal therapy. J Periodontol 2005;76:1588–1600.

35. Ward VJ. A clinical assessment of the use of the free gingival graft for correcting localized recession associated with frenal pull. J Periodontol 1974;45:78–83.

36. Addy M, Dummer PM, Hunter ML, Kingdon A, Shaw WC. A study of the association of fraenal attachment, lip coverage, and vestibular depth with plaque and gingivitis. J Periodontol 1987;58:752–757.

37. Bollen AM, Cunha-Cruz J, Bakko DW, Huang GJ, Hujoel PP. The effects of orthodontic therapy on periodontal health: A systematic review of controlled evidence. J Am Dent Assoc 2008;139:413–422.

38. Nordland WP, Tarnow DP. A classification system for loss of papillary height. J Periodontol 1998;69:1124–1126.

39. Tarnow DP, Magner AW, Fletcher P. The effect of the distance from the contact point to the crest of bone on the presence or absence of the interproximal dental papilla. J Periodontol 1992;63:995–996.

40. Coslet JG, Vanarsdall R, Weisgold A. Diagnosis and classification of delayed passive eruption of the dentogingival junction in the adult. Alpha Omegan 1977;70(3):24–28.

41. Wagenberg BD, Eskow RN, Langer B. Exposing adequate tooth structure for restorative dentistry. Int J Periodontics Restorative Dent 1989;9:322–331.

42. Deas DE, Moritz AJ, McDonnell HT, Powell CA, Mealey BL. Osseous surgery for crown lengthening: A 6-month clinical study. J Periodontol 2004;75:1288–1294.

43. Brägger U, Lauchenauer D, Lang NP. Surgical lengthening of the clinical crown. J Clin Periodontol 1992;19:58–63.

44. Goldstein M, Nasatzky E, Goultschin J, Boyan BD, Schwartz Z. Coverage of previously carious roots is as predictable a procedure as coverage of intact roots. J Periodontol 2002;73:1419–1426.

45. Orsini G, Murmura G, Artese L, Piattelli A, Piccirilli M, Caputi S. Tissue healing under provisional restorations with ovate pontics: A pilot human histological study. J Prosthet Dent 2006;96:252–257.

46. Spear FM. The use of implants and ovate pontics in the esthetic zone. Compend Contin Educ Dent 2008;29:72–74,76–80.

47. Harris RJ. Root coverage in molar recession: Report of 50 consecutive cases treated with subepithelial connective tissue grafts. J Periodontol 2003;74:703–708.

12

Regeneration

Background

Q: Define periodontal regeneration, reattachment, new attachment, and repair.

- *Periodontal regeneration:* Restoration of the lost periodontium or supporting tissues
- *Reattachment:* Reunion of the epithelium or connective tissue to the root surface or bone
- *New attachment:* Union of connective tissue or epithelium with the root surface that has been deprived of its original attachment apparatus
- *Repair:* Healing of the wound by tissue—does not fully restore architecture or function

Note that scaling and root planing and most flap surgeries heal by repair.

Q: What are the goals of regeneration?

- Regenerate new bone
- Reduce or eliminate osseous defects
- Stop attachment loss
- Stop or reduce the inflammation
- Increase tooth stability
- Recover esthetics

Q: Describe the four different cell types that can repopulate the root surface after periodontal surgery.

Melcher[1] described the four cell types as follows:

1. Long junctional epithelium: If these cells populate first, there will be no bone regeneration.
2. Gingival connective tissue cells: May lead to root resorption.
3. Bone cells: Resorption and ankylosis.
4. Periodontal ligament cells: New cementum forms perpendicular to junctional epithelium.

Melcher believed that it was important to allow selective repopulation of the wound and exclude epithelium.

Q: What factors are important for regeneration?

- Patient factors: The patient should not smoke and must have good oral hygiene.
- Inflammation should be controlled as much as possible before surgery to allow better flap reflection and suturing.
- Defect factors: The deeper, narrower, and greater number of walls, the better (Fig 12-1). Kim et al[2] found that bone regeneration averaged 1.5, 1.7, and 2.3 mm for one-, two-, and three-wall defects, respectively, with the three-wall defects being significantly different from the one-wall defects. They concluded that the number of bone walls is a critical factor determining treatment outcomes in intrabony periodontal defects.

Fig 12-1 Deep and narrow defect between the canine and the premolar.

- Factors associated with technique: Flap design and preservation of the interdental papillae are important. It is also important to perform scaling and root planing of the teeth before regeneration is performed and to minimize trauma to the flap.

Q: What is guided tissue regeneration (GTR)?

In GTR, the clinician tries to control the cells repopulating the site by placing a barrier membrane. It is used during wound healing to prevent epithelial and connective tissue growth.

Q: What is guided bone regeneration (GBR)?

GBR is similar to GTR except that a bone graft is generally used in addition to a membrane to successfully augment bone formation.

Q: What is the Misch bone density scale?

- D1: Dense cortical bone found in the anterior mandible
- D2: Thick, dense cortical bone on the crest and coarse trabecular bone within
- D3: Thin, porous cortical bone and fine trabecular bone within
- D4: Fine trabecular bone
- D5: Immature, nonmineralized bone

Bone Grafting

Q: What is the difference between osteogenetic, osteoinductive, and osteoconductive bone material?

- *Osteogenetic:* New bone formation occurs as a result of bone-forming cells contained in the graft.
- *Osteoinductive:* Bone formation is induced in the surrounding soft tissue immediately adjacent to the grafted material. An example is demineralized freeze-dried bone allograft (DFDBA).
- *Osteoconductive:* Graft material does not directly contribute to new bone formation but serves as a scaffold for bone formation by adjacent host bone. An example is freeze-dried bone allograft (FDBA).

Q: Describe the different types of graft material.

- *Autogenous graft:* Graft is transferred from one position to another within the same individual. A second surgical site is needed (eg, retromolar pad, maxillary tuberosity).
- *Allograft:* A graft between genetically dissimilar members of the same species.
- *Xenograft:* A graft from a donor of another species.
- *Alloplast:* Synthetic or inorganic implant material used as a substitute for a bone graft.

Q: Are allografts safe?

Most bone banks adhere to the guidelines of the American Association of Tissue Banks (AATB).[3] The AATB excludes collection in the following circumstances:

- Donor is from a high-risk group
- Donor tests positive for HIV
- Autopsy of the donor reveals occult disease
- Donor tests positive for bacterial contamination
- Donor and bone test positive for hepatitis B or C
- Donor tests positive for syphilis

Mellonig et al[4] found that spiked and infected bone treated with a virucidal agent inactivates HIV.

Q: What are the different applications for onlay, veneer block, and saddle grafts?

- Onlay graft: Vertical or horizontal reconstruction of bone
- Veneer block graft: Horizontal augmentation of bone
- Saddle graft: Horizontal and vertical augmentation of bone—could use a J- or L-shaped graft

Q: What is the success rate for allogenic block augmentation?

In a multicenter evaluation, Keith et al[5] found the following success rates for allogenic block grafts by region:

- Anterior maxilla: 94% (2/35 block grafts lost)
- Maxillary molar region: 100% (0 lost)
- Anterior mandible: 67% (1/3 lost)
- Mandibular molar region: 87% (5/38 lost)

Q: What is the resorption rate for block grafts?

Nissan et al[6] evaluated the outcome of ridge augmentation with cancellous freeze-dried block bone allografts in the posterior atrophic mandible followed by placement of dental implants. Horizontal augmentation was 5.6 mm and vertical augmentation was 4.3 mm. Resorption of the buccal bone averaged 0.5 mm at the time of implant placement and 0.2 mm at stage-two surgery.

McAllister and Haghighat[7] noted that augmentation with autogenous bone grafts resulted in resorption rates of 0% to 25% at implant placement and up to 60% at the time of abutment placement. The study found that barrier membranes placed with block grafts optimized ridge augmentation (in regard to graft resorption).

Q: **Describe some studies that show that bone grafting is effective.**

- In 1991, Mellonig[8] conducted a study in which 327 sites were treated with FDBA only and 176 sites were treated with FDBA and autogenous bone. The study found complete or greater than 50% bone fill in 67% of sites treated with FDBA alone and 78% of sites treated with FDBA and autogenous bone.
- The results of a 2003 meta-analysis by Reynolds et al[9] supported the following statements regarding the treatment of intrabony defects: (1) Bone grafts increase bone level, reduce crestal bone loss, increase clinical attachment level, and reduce probing depth compared with open-flap debridement (OFD) procedures. (2) Randomized controlled studies provide evidence that DFDBA supports the formation of a new attachment apparatus in intrabony defects, whereas OFD results in periodontal repair characterized primarily by the formation of a long junctional epithelial attachment.
- In a 1989 histologic evaluation of new attachment apparatus formation by Bowers et al,[10] data from 12 patients with 32 DFDBA-grafted and 25 nongrafted defects were studied. A long junctional epithelium formed along the entire length of exposed root in nongrafted sites. In contrast, grafted sites gained new attachment apparatus, new cementum, new connective tissue, and new bone.
- In 2000, Mellonig[11] conducted a human histologic evaluation of a bovine-derived bone xenograft (Bio-Oss, Geistlich) in the treatment of periodontal osseous defects. In three of the four specimens, histologic observations demonstrated new bone, new cementum, and new periodontal ligament. Grafting with a bovine-derived xenograft allows for periodontal regeneration.
- In a 1970 study of iliac transplants in periodontal therapy, Schallhorn et al[12] found that iliac grafts are effective, but they can cause external resorption, infection, and sequestra.
- Buser et al[13] carried out lateral ridge augmentation using autografts and barrier membranes in a 1996 clinical study with 40 partially edentulous patients, demonstrating that the combined application of autografts and expanded polytetrafluoroethylene (e-PTFE) membranes is a predictable surgical procedure for lateral ridge augmentation that results in a 4-mm increase of width of bone.

Although there is significant evidence acclaiming the effectiveness of bone grafting, Cortellini and Tonetti[14] did a study without regenerative materials and obtained results similar to those of studies that did use regenerative materials. A group of 45 patients received either a modified minimally invasive surgical technique (M-MIST) alone, with enamel matrix protein, or with enamel matrix protein and xenograft. Significant clinical and radiographic improvements were found when M-MIST was used with or without regenerative materials. The human body can induce regeneration of its own tissue.

Q: Is there a difference between bone graft materials (FDBA, DFDBA, and xenografts)?

Wood and Mealey[15] found that FDBA had a significantly decreased percentage of vital bone at 24.63% versus DFDBA at 38.42%. FDBA also had a significantly greater mean percentage of residual graft particles at 25.42% compared with DFDBA at 8.88%. Yukna and Vastardis,[16] on the other hand, found that FDBA stimulates faster and more substantial new bone formation than DFDBA in a monkey jaw defect model system.

A 2005 AAP position paper[17] found bone fill ranging from 1.3 to 2.6 mm when FDBA was used to treat defects. Human trials using DFDBA have demonstrated bone fill similar to that achieved with FDBA, ranging from 1.7 to 2.9 mm. Rummelhart et al[18] studied 22 defects in nine patients using DFDBA and FDBA and found no significant differences between the treatment groups.

Q: Discuss the variability in the ability of DFDBA to induce new bone formation.

The following are possible reasons for the variability in new bone formation induced by DFDBA[3]:

- Bone induction proteins are not present in sufficient quantity to produce detectable bone formation.
- Bone-inductive components of DFDBA are present but are in an inactive form.
- Some DFDBA batches are more active than others (based on content of bone-inductive factors in donor).
- Sterilization processing may be an important contributor to variability of DFDBA.
- Wide variations in commercial bone bank preparations of DFDBA exist.
- Donor age, but not sex, may also play a role.
- Particle size also appears to be an important variable in the success of DFDBA as a bone-inductive material. Particles in the range of 125 to 1,000 µm possess a higher osteogenic potential than do particles below 125 µm.

Q: Is the alloplast calcium sulfate effective?

Choi et al[19] found bone regeneration with the synthetic biomaterials amorphous calcium phosphate (ACP) and micro-macroporous biphasic calcium phosphate (MBCP) similar to that with FDBA in surgically generated three-wall intrabony defects adjacent to implants. The study concluded that FDBA is as effective as ACP and MBCP at osteoconduction.

Aimetti et al[20] evaluated whether the placement of medical-grade calcium sulfate hemihydrate in fresh extraction sockets might affect the quality of newly formed bone and influence crestal bone changes. The study found that from the crestal to the apical region of specimens treated with the alloplast, the mean percentage of lamellar bone increased from 16.4% to 43.6%, compared with 11.1% to 22.2% in unfilled specimens.

Q: Does particle size make a difference in the success of the bone graft material?

Shapoff et al[21] indicated that there was significantly decreased new bone formation associated with large-particle (1,000- to 2,000-µm) FDBA plus autogenous marrow than with small-particle (100- to 300-µm) FDBA plus autogenous marrow. In addition, large-particle FDBA plus autogenous marrow tended to display less resorption than small-particle FDBA plus autogenous marrow.

In a study by Fucini et al,[22] after reentry average bony defect fill was 1.32 mm for the small-particle (250- to 500-µm) group and 1.66 mm for the large-particle (850- to 1,000-µm) group. Different particle sizes of DFDBA showed no statistically significant difference in bony fill.

Q: Does adding tetracycline to the bone graft make it more effective?

Figure 12-2 shows a site grafted with particulate bone plus tetracycline.

Fig 12-2 Particulate bone mixed with tetracycline in a grafted site.

Drury and Yukna[23] mixed tetracycline and FDBA in experimental defects in baboons. The study found that FDBA in combination with tetracycline improves new bone formation in experimental alveolar bone defects.

A study by Masters et al[24] found only a slight difference in bone fill between a DFDBA and tetracycline group (2.27 mm) and a DFDBA only group (2.20 mm) and reported no statistically significant differences between the groups in any clinical parameters. The authors concluded that the addition of 50 mg/mL of tetracycline hydrochloride to the allograft did not result in any significant benefits.

Q: Is decortication of the bone important?

Rompen et al[25] demonstrated greater regeneration in skulls perforated with nine 0.8-mm diameter holes (172.8%) compared with skulls with an intact osseous surface (141%). De novo bone formation occurs by stimulation of the blood supply and access of bone-forming cells by cortical perforations.

Adeyemo et al[26] found no difference in terms of healing and integration of the bone graft between perforated and nonperforated recipient cortical beds.

Greenstein et al[27] did a review of the literature and found that there is inconsistent literature and inadequate clinical research to make any conclusions as to the benefits of bone decortication preceding GBR procedures.

Membranes

Q: What are some important properties of membranes?

Figure 12-3 presents properties that membranes should possess to be clinically effective.

Fig 12-3 Properties of membranes.

Q: What are the two types of membranes?

Figure 12-4 presents characteristics of the two types of membranes: resorbable and nonresorbable.

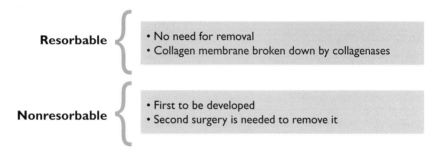

Resorbable
- No need for removal
- Collagen membrane broken down by collagenases

Nonresorbable
- First to be developed
- Second surgery is needed to remove it

Fig 12-4 Characteristics of resorbable and nonresorbable membranes.

Q: Is there a difference in treatment outcome between resorbable and nonresorbable membranes?

In a 2010 study, Merli et al[28] randomly allocated patients into two treatment groups—resorbable and titanium-reinforced membranes. Each group had 11 patients needing vertical bone augmentation. The study noted no statistically significant difference in bone loss between the two groups at either 1 or 3 years. At the 3-year mark, the resorbable membrane group lost an average of 0.55 mm of bone, while patients in the nonresorbable barrier group had an average of 0.53 mm of bone loss.

In a 1997 study, Caffesse et al[29] randomly placed patients in resorbable and nonresorbable membrane groups. In the nonresorbable group, the membrane was removed at 6 weeks. The study found no differences between the groups. The study concluded that, in terms of treating grade II furcations and intrabony defects, the resorbable membrane and the nonresorbable e-PTFE membrane were equally effective.

In a 1998 study, Laurell et al[30] concluded that there is no difference between resorbable and nonresorbable membranes. The study came to this conclusion by evaluating studies presented during the previous 20 years on the surgical treatment of intrabony defects. The authors examined treatment outcomes of OFD, bone replacement grafts, and GTR.

Q: What is the effect of membrane exposure?

Figure 12-5 shows an exposed resorbable membrane during a socket grafting procedure.

Fig 12-5 *(a)* Exposed resorbable membrane after socket grafting. *(b)* The exposed resorbable membrane covered with a free gingival graft.

Machtei[31] found that nonresorbable and resorbable membrane exposure during healing had a minimal effect on GTR around natural teeth. However, it had a significant negative impact on GBR around dental implants; exposed membranes had 0.56 mm and submerged membranes had 3.01 mm of bone regeneration around implants.

An analysis by De Sanctis et al[32] found that exposed areas of membranes had bacterial colonization in all the microscopic fields. Although no bacteria-positive field was observed in the most apical portion of the membranes, the middle portion of many of the membranes (16 of 39 [41%]) demonstrated microbial colonization.

Q: How is membrane exposure managed postoperatively?

Figure 12-6 presents the steps involved in postoperative management of membrane exposure. Note that if a nonresorbable membrane is exposed, it should be removed in 4 to 6 weeks to prevent a negative effect on bone regeneration.

Fig 12-6 Postoperative management of membrane exposure.

Q: Should antibiotics be given to patients when a membrane is placed?

The patient should take antibiotics for 1 week and rinse with 12% chlorhexidine for 12 weeks after GBR to reduce postoperative infection and ensure optimal clinical results.[33]

In a study by Nowzari et al,[34] the experimental group received Augmentin (GlaxoSmithKline) and GTR (nonresorbable membrane) while the control group only had GTR (nonresorbable membrane). A significantly higher gain in mean probing attachment was found at 6 months in the test group (36.5% of potential gain) compared with the control group (22.4% of potential gain). When the membranes were removed, significantly fewer organisms were found in the test group (52.2×10^6) compared with the control group (488.6×10^6).

Q: Is there a difference between cross-linked and non–cross-linked membranes?

Tal et al[35] found that although both cross-linked and non–cross-linked membranes degraded when exposed to the oral environment, both membranes were resistant to tissue degradation and preserved continuity throughout the study.

When membranes were prematurely exposed, Moses et al[36] found bony defect healing to be significantly higher in the cross-linked Ossix (OraPharma) group than in the other two groups (non–cross-linked Bio-Gide [Geistlich] and Gore-Tex [W. L. Gore]). They also found statistically similar defect reduction in the patients with prematurely exposed Ossix membranes and those with unexposed membranes.

Bornstein et al[37] found that the cross-linked membrane placed in dog mandibles for bone regeneration had a limited beneficial effect when healing was uneventful. They compared the cross-linked membrane to a collagen membrane.

Q: What is the difference between Bio-Gide and BioMend membranes?

Figure 12-7 presents the characteristics of Bio-Gide and BioMend (Zimmer) membranes.

Bio-Gide	BioMend
• Non–cross-linked, porcine-derived collagen (type I and type III). • Resorption time varies depending on a number of factors, including but not limited to the surgical site, occurrence of dehiscence, loading, type of fixation, and the patient.	• Bovine achilles tendon collagen (type I). • BioMend collagen membrane is absorbed in approximately 8 weeks. • BioMend Extend collagen membrane is absorbed in approximately 18 weeks.

Fig 12-7 Bio-Gide versus BioMend.

Q: What is the technique for membrane placement?

1. Slightly divergent vertical incisions are initiated at proximal line angles one tooth anterior and one tooth posterior to the treated tooth/area. They should extend apical to the mucogingival junction.
2. A horizontal incision is made, and a full-thickness flap is carried out to expose the entire perimeter of the dehiscence.
3. Degranulation is performed.
4. The membrane should cover 3 mm of bone beyond the defect margins, and the apical margin of the membrane should be 2 to 3 mm apical to the flap margin.

Q: **What are tacks and screws used for?**

Tacks are used to stabilize the membrane.[38] Screws are used for bone stabilization. It is important to place at least two screws to prevent rotation.

Considerations for Regeneration

Q: **What are some ideal anatomical considerations when regenerating bone?**

Tonetti et al[39] found greater linear gains in deeper pockets. The study also found that, at an angle of 25 degrees or less (bony wall to long axis of the tooth), there was 1.6 mm more attachment than in defects with an angle of 37 degrees or more.

Laurell et al[30] compared OFD alone and OFD plus DFDBA, FDBA, or autogenous GTR. The study found that the intrabony defect has to be at least 4 mm deep to benefit from GTR procedures.

Q: **How does GTR compare to OFD?**

Figure 12-8 presents studies comparing GTR and OFD.

Laurell et al[30] (1998)	Murphy and Gunsolley[40] (2003)	Needleman et al[41] (2006)
• This article reviews studies presented during the last 20 years on the surgical treatment of intrabony defects. Treatments include OFD; OFD plus DFDBA, FDBA, or autogenous bone; and GTR. • GTR resulted in significant pocket reduction, clinical attachment gain of 4.2 mm, and bone fill averaging 3.2 mm versus OFD with clinical attachment gain of 1.5 mm and bone fill of 1.1 mm.	• This review's aim was to compare GTR in control patients and patients with periodontal osseous defects. • Patients who received GTR had a gain of clinical attachment and a reduction in probing depth compared with those receiving OFD. • Physical barriers and bone replacement grafts placed together have been shown to enhance clinical outcome in furcation defects. • Coverage of the barrier with a coronally advanced flap is associated with a better outcome.	• The study compared GTR and OFD in the treatment of periodontal infrabony defects using the Cochrane Oral Health Group Trials Register, MEDLINE, and EMBASE up to April 2004. • Although there is a marked variability between studies, improved attachment gain, less increase in gingival recession, more gain in hard tissue, and reduced pocket depth were observed with GTR compared with OFD at reentry surgery.

Fig 12-8 Studies comparing GTR and OFD.

Q: What is distraction osteogenesis?

Distraction osteogenesis is based on the concept that new bone fills a gap created when two pieces of bone are separated slowly under tension. It is important to have a minimum of 6 to 7 mm of bone height above vital structures. The ridge defect should be greater than 3 to 4 mm, and the edentulous ridge span should be three or more missing teeth.[7] Figure 12-9 presents the phases of distraction osteogenesis.

Latency	**Distraction**	**Consolidation**
7 days for soft tissue healing	Two pieces of bone undergo separation at a rate of 1 mm per day	Allows bone regeneration in the created space

Fig 12-9 Distraction osteogenesis phases.

Q: What are the options for horizontal ridge augmentation?

- Bone and membrane (Fig 12-10): Fuggazotto[42] completed 289 ridge augmentation surgeries. Various configurations of Gore-Tex membranes were used in addition to various nonautogenous particulate materials. Of the 289 augmented ridges, 279 had adequate regenerated hard tissues for implant placement in ideal prosthetic positions. The horizontally augmented ridges had a success rate of 97%.

Fig 12-10 (a) Allograft material placed for horizontal augmentation. (b) Membrane placed over the allograft for horizontal augmentation.

- Autogenous block graft (eg, tuberosity, chin, and lateral ramus).
- Ridge splitting (Fig 12-11): When doing the procedure, it is important to prevent fracture of the buccal plate. Sethi and Kaus[43] performed a 5-year study evaluating 449 implants placed in maxillary ridges expanded by the ridge-split technique. The study revealed a survival rate of 97%. According to McAllister and Haghighat,[7] the avoidance of a separate donor site with the ridge-split technique, whether it uses particulate, block graft, or GBR, and its associated reduced treatment time and morbidity represent its primary advantage compared with other lateral augmentation techniques.

Fig 12-11 *(a)* Ridge split with direction indicators. *(b)* Ridge split with implants placed.

- Distraction osteogenesis: Laster et al[44] treated nine patients with distraction osteogenesis, increasing the alveolar width from 4 to 6 mm. Of the 21 implants placed, 20 implants successfully osseointegrated. After 12 months' follow-up, no marginal bone resorption was observed. They listed soft tissue expansion, high dimensional stability, reduced treatment time, and the avoidance of a graft as the advantages of horizontal distraction compared with block grafting.
- Block allograft: Because allograft is not living bone, it must be hydrated, and air bubbles must be removed. Nissan et al[45] did a study on 40 patients (83 implants) with 60 cancellous freeze-dried bone block allografts. The study had an average percentage of newly formed bone of 33% and implant survival of 98.8%. In a two-stage implant placement procedure, cancellous bone block allograft is osteoconductive and biocompatible, allowing new bone formation following augmentation of extremely atrophic anterior maxillae.

Esposito et al[46] conducted a systematic review and observed no statistically significant differences when comparing various horizontal augmentation techniques.

Q: What are the options for vertical ridge augmentation?

- Bone and membrane (GBR with the possibility of using pins): Simion et al[47] performed a study in which vertical augmentation was performed in six different surgical sites. Five patients received 15 conical Brånemark-type implants that protruded 4 to 7 mm from the bone crest, and miniscrews were placed distally to the implants. The miniscrews and implants were enclosed with a titanium-reinforced membrane. There was vertical augmentation of 3 to 4 mm, and the retrieved miniscrews were in contact with bone based on histology. Vertical augmentation with GBR is more technique sensitive than horizontal augmentation.
- Sinus elevation (discussed in chapter 13).
- Onlay graft: Barone and Covani[48] found that the success rate of block grafts was very good. They found a very low rate of resorption both clinically and radiographically following bone graft and implant placement and concluded that grafts from the anterosuperior edge of the iliac wing are a "promising treatment" in cases of severe maxillary atrophy.
- Distraction osteogenesis: Esposito et al[46] found that distraction osteogenesis (more than any other technique) permits simultaneous horizontal and vertical augmentation.

Esposito et al[46] found in a systematic review that there can be many complications associated with vertical augmentation, and as a result, short implants may be a better option in patients with resorbed mandibles.

Vertical augmentation is difficult because it is challenging to achieve fixation, and there is a high resorption rate.

Socket Grafting

Q: What is socket grafting or ridge preservation?

After extraction of the tooth, it is important to maintain the dimensions of the ridge. Placing a bone graft into the socket (Fig 12-12) allows for this preservation, especially in the esthetic zone.

Fig 12-12 (a) Socket preservation with allograft and resorbable membrane. (b) Membrane sutured over the allograft.

Q: Describe the healing that occurs after tooth extraction.

Amler et al[49] found that after extraction, a blood clot filled the socket. After 7 days, granulation tissue filled the socket. Collagen replaced the granulation tissue and bone formation began at the base and around the extraction socket after 20 days. Bone filled about two-thirds of the socket at 5 weeks. It took 24 to 35 days for the epithelium, which grew progressively as it enveloped granulation, debris, and bone particles, to completely cover the extraction socket. At all stages, bone regeneration began at the apex and outside of the socket, progressing gradually toward its center and the crest of bone.[50]

After socket grafting, first a blood clot forms, then a few days after grafting, the first phase of the graft material dissolves. Nutrient canals and osteoblasts invade the graft, and maturation occurs.

Q: Is socket grafting effective?

In a meta-analysis, Vignoletti et al[51] found vertical and horizontal contraction of the alveolar bone crest to be less in patients who had received socket preservation. Test and control sites had a difference of 1.47 mm in bone height. The meta-analysis concluded that socket preservation limits vertical and horizontal dimensional changes after a tooth has been extracted.

McAllister and Haghighat[7] noted that bone regeneration could occur without socket grafting in extraction sockets with intact bony walls, and therefore socket grafting at the time of extraction may not always be beneficial. They cited studies in which the healing processes of socket grafts were altered when various bone grafting materials were used to preserve the alveolar ridge and socket dimensions.

A recent randomized clinical trial[52] found that implants placed into grafted sites displayed a clinical performance comparable to that of implants positioned in nongrafted sites with respect to implant survival and marginal bone loss. Yet grafted sites allowed for fewer augmentation surgeries and placement of larger implants.

Q: When should implants be placed after socket preservation?

Beck and Mealey[53] found no significant differences in the amount of new bone growth of the grafted allograft bone at 3 versus 6 months following extraction and ridge preservation. Therefore, the study did not support waiting longer periods of time following extraction and ridge preservation to permit bone regeneration.

Note that it may be prudent to look at other factors (eg, number of bony walls, angle of the defect, and age of the patient) to determine the amount of time to wait before implant placement.

Growth Factors

Q: What are the benefits and drawbacks of using growth factors for bone regeneration?[54]

The advantages and disadvantages of using growth factors for bone regeneration are shown in Fig 12-13.

+	−
• Excellent wound healing • Bone induction and chemotactic effect • Decreased need for autogenous bone • Decreased surgical time and thus less trauma to the patient • Better tissue regeneration	• Higher cost • New technologic advancement that needs to be developed over time • Greater swelling

Fig 12-13 Advantages and disadvantages of using growth factors for bone regeneration.

Q: What is enamel matrix derivative (EMD) and is it effective?

EMD is derived from porcine teeth, and it has a protein that mimics the matrix proteins that induce cementogenesis. It is a tissue-healing modulator that mimics events that occur during root development and helps stimulate periodontal regeneration.
Studies on EMD include the following:

• Froum et al[55] found that EMD use resulted in statistically larger gains in clinical attachment level and decreased probing depth.
• In a meta-analysis, Koop et al[56] found that EMD is as effective as resorbable membranes in the treatment of intrabony defects. EMD and a coronally advanced flap is as effective as a connective tissue graft.
• Esposito et al[57] found that EMD significantly improved probing attachment levels by 1.1 mm and pocket depth reduction by 0.9 mm when compared with a control, although they stated that the actual clinical advantages of using EMD were not certain. There were no findings of differences between GTR and EMD with the exception of significantly more postoperative complications in the GTR group.

- Rösing et al[58] treated 16 patients with chronic periodontitis who had greater than 6-mm defects using a split-mouth design. The control sites received a placebo, and the test sites received the EMD solution. EMD did not impact or improve clinical and radiographic parameters compared with the placebo.
- Giannobile and Somerman[59] found that clinical attachment level gain and reduction of pocket depth have been promoted with the use of EMD in osseous defects. Compared with control procedures (usually OFD), EMD has shown superior results with great consistency.

Q: Describe the importance of bone morphogenetic proteins (BMPs).

BMP-2 and BMP-7 (osteogenic protein 1), which are glycoproteins and osteoinductive, start a cycle of cellular events resulting in differentiation of cells into phenotypes involved in periodontal regeneration. They enhance bone and cementum formation. In a 1994 study, Ripamonti et al[60] made acute defects in baboons and applied BMP to the experimental group. They found that the experimental group had 2.5 times more bone and cementum height than the controls. A review by King and Cochran[61] found that a number of studies have demonstrated the potential for BMPs to increase periodontal regeneration. The effects of BMPs are influenced by root surface conditioning, occlusal loading, dosage, and carrier systems.

Q: What is platelet-derived growth factor (PDGF) and what does it do?

PDGF is derived from platelets, macrophages, and osteoblasts. It stimulates DNA and protein synthesis and regulates cell growth and division. Kaigler et al[62] suggest that PDGF in combination with osteoconductive matrices, based on clinical results of its use in various periodontal and peri-implant applications, could potentially come into routine use.

Fagan et al[63] noted that when FDBA, recombinant human PDGF (rhPDGF), and a titanium-reinforced membrane were placed for implant site augmentation, hard tissue augmentation was histologically apparent. Soft tissue was also augmented after pediculated connective tissue was rinsed with rhPDGF.

Q: What is growth factor–enhanced matrix?

Growth factor–enhanced matrix (GEM 21S, Osteohealth) combines rhPDGF and β-tricalcium phosphate (β-TCP), which mix and are released into the surrounding environment after implantation. rhPDGF then binds to specific cell surface receptors on the target cells, initiating a cascade of intracellular signaling pathways. rhPDGF-induced intracellular events lead to directed cell migration or chemotaxis and cell proliferation or mitogenesis of osteoblasts, periodontal ligament fibroblasts, and cementoblasts.[64]

In 11 clinical centers, Nevins et al[65] performed surgical treatment on 180 patients with a 4-mm or greater intrabony periodontal defect. Patients were randomly placed into one of three treatment groups: (1) β-TCP + 0.3 mg/mL rhPDGF-BB in buffer, (2) β-TCP + 1.0 mg/mL rhPDGF-BB in buffer; and (3) β-TCP + buffer (active control). At 3 months, clinical attachment gain was significantly greater for group 1 (3.8 mm) compared with group 3 (3.3 mm). Group 1 had greater defect fill (57% versus 18%) and greater linear bone gain (2.6 versus 0.9 mm) than group 3 at 6 months.

Q: **Which growth factors have the US Food and Drug Administration (FDA) cleared for periodontal regeneration?**

EMD and PDGF have been cleared by the FDA for periodontal regeneration; BMP-2 has FDA clearance for bone augmentation.[66]

Miscellaneous

Q: **Does tooth vitality affect regenerative outcomes in intrabony defects?**

Cortellini and Tonetti[67] demonstrated that deep intrabony defects do not negatively influence tooth vitality. They also found that the healing response of deep intrabony defects treated with GTR therapy is not negatively affected by root canal therapy.

Q: **How does hypermobility affect regeneration?**

Cortellini et al[68] found that severe hypermobility can negatively impact the clinical outcome of regeneration.

Q: **Does demineralization of the root surface improve regeneration?**

It was believed that exposure of the collagen in the dentinal matrix would facilitate adhesion of the blood clot to the root. However, in five out of six citric acid–treated specimens, Stahl and Froum[69] found no evidence suggesting that citric acid applications either initiated or accelerated cementogenesis or functional connective tissue attachment at root surfaces previously exposed to periodontal pockets. Moreover, a meta-analysis performed by Mariotti[70] on 28 clinical trials did not show any significant effects of acid root treatment on attachment level gains or probing depth. Evidence to date suggests that the use of citric acid, tetracycline, or ethylenediaminetetraacetic acid (EDTA) to modify the root surface provides no clinically significant benefit to regeneration in patients with chronic periodontitis.

Q: How does smoking affect regeneration?

Tonetti et al[71] performed a retrospective study investigating the influence of cigarette smoking on the healing response after GTR in deep defects. Non-smokers gained significantly more probing attachment level (5.2 mm) than smokers (2.1 mm).

Rosen et al[72] conducted a study on DFDBA in intrabony defects. At 1 year posttreatment, significant reductions in mean probing depth were observed for nonsmokers (3.8 mm) and smokers (3.0 mm). However, when relative improvements in clinical measures were compared at the 1- and 2- to 5-year follow-ups, nonsmokers were found to exhibit significantly better treatment effects. Compared to pretreatment findings, there were changes in progress detected for the clinical attachment level at the 1-year evaluation (29.2% for smokers and 42.5% for nonsmokers).

Stavropoulos et al[73] examined 47 intrabony defects in 32 patients treated by means of polylactic acid/citric acid ester copolymer resorbable membranes. Smokers had less pocket reduction than nonsmokers (4.5 ± 0.7 versus 5.5 ± 0.7 mm, respectively), which resulted in greater residual pocket depth in smokers compared with nonsmokers (3.6 ± 1.0 versus 3.4 ± 1.1 mm).

Q: How can researchers measure regeneration?

- Histology (many believe this is the only way)
- Radiographic analysis
- Probing

References

1. Melcher AH. On the repair potential of periodontal tissues. J Periodontol 1976;47:256–260.
2. Kim CS, Choi SH, Chai JK, et al. Periodontal repair in surgically created intrabony defects in dogs: Influence of the number of bone walls on healing response. J Periodontol 2004;75:229–235.
3. Committee on Research, Science and Therapy of the American Academy of Periodontology. Tissue banking of bone allografts used in periodontal regeneration. J Periodontol 2001;72:834–838.
4. Mellonig JT, Prewett AB, Moyer MP. HIV inactivation in a bone allograft. J Periodontol 1992;63:979–983.
5. Keith JD Jr, Petrungaro P, Leonetti JA et al. Clinical and histologic evaluation of a mineralized block allograft: Results from the developmental period (2001–2004). Int J Periodontics Restorative Dent 2006;26:321–327.

6. Nissan J, Ghelfan O, Mardinger O, Calderon S, Chaushu G. Efficacy of cancellous block allograft augmentation prior to implant placement in the posterior atrophic mandible. Clin Implant Dent Relat Res 2011;13:279–285.

7. McAllister BS, Haghighat K. Bone augmentation techniques. J Periodontol 2007;78:377–396.

8. Mellonig JT. Freeze-dried bone allografts in periodontal reconstructive surgery. Dent Clin North Am 1991;35:505–520.

9. Reynolds MA, Aichelmann-Reidy ME, Branch-Mays GL, Gunsolley JC. The efficacy of bone re-placement grafts in the treatment of periodontal osseous defects. A systematic review. Ann Periodontol 2003;8:227–265.

10. Bowers GM, Chadroff B, Carnevale R, et al. Histologic evaluation of new attachment apparatus formation in humans. Part III. J Periodontol 1989;60:683–693.

11. Mellonig JT. Human histologic evaluation of a bovine-derived bone xenograft in the treatment of periodontal osseous defects. Int J Periodontics Restorative Dent 2000;20:19–29.

12. Schallhorn RG, Hiatt WH, Boyce W. Iliac transplants in periodontal therapy. J Periodontol 1970;41:566–580.

13. Buser D, Dula K, Hirt HP, Schenk RK. Lateral ridge augmentation using autografts and bar-rier membranes: A clinical study with 40 partially edentulous patients. J Oral Maxillofac Surg 1996;54:420–433.

14. Cortellini P, Tonetti MS. Clinical and radiographic outcomes of the modified minimally invasive surgical technique with and without regenerative materials: A randomized-controlled trial in intra-bony defects. J Clin Periodontol 2011;38:365–373.

15. Wood RA, Mealey BL. Histologic comparison of healing after tooth extraction with ridge pres-ervation using mineralized versus demineralized freeze-dried bone allograft. J Periodontol 2012;83:329–336.

16. Yukna RA, Vastardis S. Comparative evaluation of decalcified and non-decalcified freeze-dried bone allografts in rhesus monkeys. I. Histologic findings. J Periodontol 2005;76:57–65.

17. Wang HL, Greenwell H, Fiorellini J, et al; Research, Science and Therapy Committee of the American Academy of Periodontology. Position paper: Periodontal regeneration. J Periodontol 2005;76:1601–1622.

18. Rummelhart JM, Mellonig JT, Gray JL, Towle HJ. A comparison of freeze-dried bone allograft and demineralized freeze-dried bone allograft in human periodontal osseous defects. J Periodontol 1989;60:655–663.

19. Choi JY, Jung UW, Lee IS, Kim CS, Lee YK, Choi SH. Resolution of surgically created three-wall intrabony defects in implants using three different biomaterials: An in vivo study. Clin Oral Im-plants Res 2011;22:343–348.

20. Aimetti M, Romano F, Griga FB, Godio L. Clinical and histologic healing of human extraction sockets filled with calcium sulfate. Int J Oral Maxillofac Implants 2009;24:902–909.

21. Shapoff CA, Bowers GM, Levy B, Mellonig JT, Yukna RA. The effect of particle size on the os-teogenic activity of composite grafts of allogeneic freeze-dried bone and autogenous marrow. J Periodontol 1980;51:625–630.

22. Fucini SE, Quintero G, Gher ME, Black BS, Richardson AC. Small versus large particles of de-mineralized freeze-dried bone allografts in human intrabony periodontal defects. J Periodontol 1993;64:844–847.

23. Drury GI, Yukna RA. Histologic evaluation of combining tetracycline and allogeneic freeze-dried bone on bone regeneration in experimental defects in baboons. J Periodontol 1991;62:652–658.

24. Masters LB, Mellonig JT, Brunsvold MA, Nummikoski PV. A clinical evaluation of demineralized freeze-dried bone allograft in combination with tetracycline in the treatment of periodontal os-seous defects. J Periodontol 1996;67:770–781.

25. Rompen EH, Biewer R, Vanheusden A, Zahedi S, Nusgens B. The influence of cortical perforations and of space filling with peripheral blood on the kinetics of guided bone generation. A compara-tive histometric study in the rat. Clin Oral Implants Res 1999;10:85–94.

26. Adeyemo WL, Reuther T, Bloch W, et al. Influence of host periosteum and recipient bed perfora-tion on the healing of onlay mandibular bone graft: An experimental pilot study in the sheep. Oral Maxillofac Surg 2008;12:19–28.

27. Greenstein G, Greenstein B, Cavallaro J, Tarnow D. The role of bone decortication in enhancing the results of guided bone regeneration: A literature review. J Periodontol 2009;80:175–189.

28. Merli M, Lombardini F, Esposito M. Vertical ridge augmentation with autogenous bone grafts 3 years after loading: Resorbable barriers versus titanium-reinforced barriers. A randomized con-trolled clinical trial. Int J Oral Maxillofac Implants 2010;25:801–807.

29. Caffesse RG, Mota LF, Quiñones CR, Morrison EC. Clinical comparison of resorbable and non-resorbable barriers for guided periodontal tissue regeneration. J Clin Periodontol 1997;24:747–752.

30. Laurell L, Gottlow J, Zybutz M, Persson R. Treatment of intrabony defects by different surgical procedures. A literature review. J Periodontol 1998;69:303–313.

31. Machtei EE. The effect of membrane exposure on the outcome of regenerative procedures in humans: A meta-analysis. J Periodontol 2001;72:512–516.

32. De Sanctis M, Zucchelli G, Clauser C. Bacterial colonization of bioabsorbable barrier material and periodontal regeneration. J Periodontol 1996;67:1193–1200.

33. Villar CC, Cochran DL. Regeneration of periodontal tissues: Guided tissue regeneration. Dent Clin North Am 2010;54:73–92.

34. Nowzari H, Matian F, Slots J. Periodontal pathogens on polytetrafluoroethylene membrane for guided tissue regeneration inhibit healing. J Clin Periodontol 1995;22:469–474.

35. Tal H, Kozlovsky A, Artzi Z, Nemcovsky CE, Moses O. Cross-linked and non-cross-linked collagen barrier membranes disintegrate following surgical exposure to the oral environment: A histological study in the cat. Clin Oral Implants Res 2008;19:760–766.

36. Moses O, Pitaru S, Artzi Z, Nemcovsky CE. Healing of dehiscence-type defects in implants placed together with different barrier membranes: A comparative clinical study. Clin Oral Implants Res 2005;16:210–219.

37. Bornstein MM, Bosshardt D, Buser D. Effect of two different bioabsorbable collagen membranes on guided bone regeneration: A comparative histomorphometric study in the dog mandible. J Periodontol 2007;78:1943–1953.

38. Block MS. Preserving alveolar ridge anatomy following tooth removal in conjunction with delayed implant placement. Atlas Oral Maxillofac Surg Clin North Am 1999;7:61–77.

39. Tonetti MS, Pini-Prato G, Cortellini P. Periodontal regeneration of human intrabony defects. IV. Determinants of healing response. J Periodontol 1993;64:934–940.

40. Murphy KG, Gunsolley JC. Guided tissue regeneration for the treatment of periodontal intrabony and furcation defects. A systematic review. Ann Periodontol 2003;8:266–302.

41. Needleman IG, Worthington HV, Giedrys-Leeper E, Tucker RJ. Guided tissue regeneration for periodontal infra-bony defects. Cochrane Database Syst Rev 2006;(2):CD001724.

42. Fugazzotto PA. Report of 302 consecutive ridge augmentation procedures: Technical considerations and clinical results. Int J Oral Maxillofac Implants 1998;13:358–368.

43. Sethi A, Kaus T. Maxillary ridge expansion with simultaneous implant placement: 5-year results of an ongoing clinical study. Int J Oral Maxillofac Implants 2000;15:491–499.

44. Laster Z, Rachmiel A, Jensen OT. Alveolar width distraction osteogenesis for early implant placement. J Oral Maxillofac Surg 2005;63:1724–1730.

45. Nissan J, Marilena V, Gross O, Mardinger O, Chaushu G. Histomorphometric analysis following augmentation of the anterior atrophic maxilla with cancellous bone block allograft. Int J Oral Maxillofac Implants 2012;27:84–89.

46. Esposito M, Grusovin MG, Felice P, Karatzopoulos G, Worthington HV, Coulthard P. The efficacy of horizontal and vertical bone augmentation procedures for dental implants—A Cochrane systematic review. Eur J Oral Implantol 2009;2:167–184.

47. Simion M, Trisi P, Piattelli A. Vertical ridge augmentation using a membrane technique associated with osseointegrated implants. Int J Periodontics Restorative Dent 1994;14:496–511.

48. Barone A, Covani U. Maxillary alveolar ridge reconstruction with nonvascularized autogenous block bone: Clinical results. J Oral Maxillofac Surg 2007;65:2039–2046.

49. Amler MH, Johnson PL, Salman I. Histological and histochemical investigation of human alveolar socket healing in undisturbed extraction wounds. J Am Dent Assoc 1960;61:32–44.

50. Steiner GG, Francis W, Burrell R, Kallet MP, Steiner DM, Macias R. The healing socket and socket regeneration. Compend Contin Educ Dent 2008;29:114–116,118,120–124.

51. Vignoletti F, Matesanz P, Rodrigo D, Figuero E, Martin C, Sanz M. Surgical protocols for ridge preservation after tooth extraction. A systematic review. Clin Oral Implants Res 2012;23(suppl 5):22–38.

52. Barone A, Orlando B, Cingano L, Marconcini S, Derchi G, Covani U. A randomized clinical trial to evaluate and compare implants placed in augmented versus non-augmented extraction sockets: 3-year results. J Periodontol 2012;83:836–846.

53. Beck TM, Mealey BL. Histologic analysis of healing after tooth extraction with ridge preservation using mineralized human bone allograft. J Periodontol 2010;81:1765–1772.

54. Jovanovic SA. Out of the vein or out of the bottle? Presented at the 98th Annual Meeting of the American Academy of Periodontology, Los Angeles, 2 Oct 2012.

55. Froum S, Lemler J, Horowitz R, Davidson B. The use of enamel matrix derivative in the treatment of periodontal osseous defects: A clinical decision tree based on biologic principles of regeneration. Int J Periodontics Restorative Dent 2001;21:437–449.

56. Koop R, Merheb J, Quirynen M. Periodontal regeneration with enamel matrix derivative in reconstructive periodontal therapy: A systematic review. J Periodontol 2012;83:707–720.

57. Esposito M, Grusovin MG, Papanikolaou N, Coulthard P, Worthington HV. Enamel matrix derivative (Emdogain[R]) for periodontal tissue regeneration in intrabony defects. Cochrane Database Syst Rev 2009;(4):CD003875.

58. Rösing CK, Aass AM, Mavropoulos A, Gjermo P. Clinical and radiographic effects of enamel matrix derivative in the treatment of intrabony periodontal defects: A 12-month longitudinal placebo-controlled clinical trial in adult periodontitis patients. J Periodontol 2005;76:129–133.

59. Giannobile WV, Somerman MJ. Growth and amelogenin-like factors in periodontal wound healing. A systematic review. Ann Periodontol 2003;8:193–204.

60. Ripamonti U, Heliotis M, van den Heever B, Reddi AH. Bone morphogenetic proteins induce periodontal regeneration in the baboon (*Papio ursinus*). J Periodontal Res 1994;29:439–445 [erratum 1995;30:149–151].

61. King GN, Cochran DL. Factors that modulate the effects of bone morphogenetic protein-induced periodontal regeneration: A critical review. J Periodontol 2002;73:925–936.

62. Kaigler D, Avila G, Wisner-Lynch L, et al. Platelet-derived growth factor applications in periodontal and peri-implant bone regeneration. Expert Opin Biol Ther 2011;11:375–385.

63. Fagan MC, Miller RE, Lynch SE, Kao RT. Simultaneous augmentation of hard and soft tissues for implant site preparation using recombinant human platelet-derived growth factor: A human case report. Int J Periodontics Restorative Dent 2008;28:37–43.

64. The Science of rhPDGF-BB: Scientifically Proven Mechanism of Action. Osteohealth website. http://www.osteohealth.com/TheScienceofrhPDGFBB.aspx. Accessed 16 October 2012.

65. Nevins M, Giannobile WV, McGuire MK, et al. Platelet-derived growth factor stimulates bone fill and rate of attachment level gain: Results of a large multicenter randomized controlled trial. J Periodontol 2005;76:2205–2215.

66. Bashutski JD, Wang HL. Biologic agents to promote periodontal regeneration and bone augmentation. Clin Adv Periodontics 2011;1:80–87.

67. Cortellini P, Tonetti MS. Evaluation of the effect of tooth vitality on regenerative outcomes in infrabony defects. J Clin Periodontol 2001;28:672–679.

68. Cortellini P, Labriola A, Tonetti MS. Regenerative periodontal therapy in intrabony defects: State of the art. Minerva Stomatol 2007;56:519–539.

69. Stahl SS, Froum SJ. Human clinical and histologic repair responses following the use of citric acid in periodontal therapy. J Periodontol 1977;48:261–266.

70. Mariotti A. Efficacy of chemical root surface modifiers in the treatment of periodontal disease. A systematic review. Ann Periodontol 2003;8:205–226.

71. Tonetti MS, Pini-Prato G, Cortellini P. Effect of cigarette smoking on periodontal healing following GTR in infrabony defects. A preliminary retrospective study. J Clin Periodontol 1995;22:229–234.

72. Rosen PS, Marks MH, Reynolds MA. Influence of smoking on long-term clinical results of intrabony defects treated with regenerative therapy. J Periodontol 1996;67:1159–1163.

73. Stavropoulos A, Mardas N, Herrero F, Karring T. Smoking affects the outcome of guided tissue regeneration with bioresorbable membranes: A retrospective analysis of intrabony defects. J Clin Periodontol 2004;31:945–950.

Implants

Background

Q: Which classification is important to take into account before placing implants?

Lekholm and Zarb[1] classified the jaws according to bone quantity and quality (Fig 13-1).

Bone quantity	Bone quality
• A: The alveolar ridge is intact • B: Moderate ridge resorption has occurred • C: Advanced residual ridge resorption has occurred • D: Some resorption of the basal bone has begun • E: Extreme resorption of the basal bone has transpired	• 1: Entire jaw is cortical bone • 2: Thick cortical bone surrounds a core of dense trabecular bone • 3: Thin layer of cortical bone surrounds a core of dense trabecular bone • 4: Thin layer of cortical bone surrounds low-density trabecular bone

Fig 13-1 Lekholm and Zarb classification[1] of bone quantity and quality.

Q: What are the criteria for successful dental implants?

Following are criteria for a successful outcome with implant placement[2,3]:

- The implant is immobile (less than 1-mm mobility in any direction) and functioning.
- No radiographic evidence of radiolucency.
- Vertical bone loss is less than 0.2 mm annually following the implant's first year of service.
- Implant has an absence of persistent and/or irreversible signs.
- Patient and clinician satisfaction.
- The hard and soft tissues are healthy.
- A trained and experienced surgeon.
- Maintenance and oral hygiene.
- Management of the soft tissues.
- A well-designed restoration.

Q: How much remodeling can be expected after an implant is placed?

Adell et al[4] found an average of 1.5 mm of marginal bone loss during healing and the first year after connection of the partial denture. Subsequently, 0.1 mm was lost annually.

Q: What are some factors that affect implant success?

- Bone quantity and quality
- Surgical technique (eg, overheating of the bone and torque forces)
- Implant length and width
- Smoking
- Amount of plaque
- Occlusion (avoiding nonaxial forces, cantilevers, and lateral excursive movements)
- Lack of keratinized attached gingiva
- Anatomy (lingual concavity, mental nerve, sinus location)

Q: What factors lead to implant failure?

- Infection (bacterial contamination and increased inflammation)
- Fracture
- Impaired healing
- Improper implant preparation (eg, overheating or overpreparation) (Fig 13-2)
- Improper mechanical stability following insertion of the implant (mobility)
- Premature loading of the implant
- Pain

Fig 13-2 Implant placed too buccal (improper implant preparation).

Q: Does location of the implant in the maxilla or mandible have an impact on implant success?

Cochran[3] found that mandibular implants have superior outcomes compared with maxillary implants. One reason for this variability is the difference in the quality of the bone. Areas with cortical bone (anterior mandible) have greater success rates compared with areas with reduced bone quality (posterior maxilla).

Becker et al[5] found collective success rates in mandibular and maxillary anterior segments to be greater than those at molar sites (91.5% in the mandible, 82.9% in the maxilla). Bone quality and quantity may be associated with differences in outcomes between anterior and posterior locations.

Q: What are contraindications to implant therapy?

Figure 13-3 presents contraindications to implant therapy.

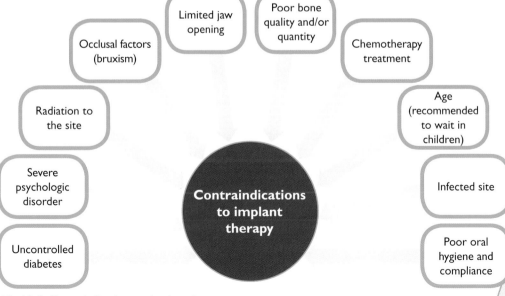

Fig 13-3 Contraindications to implant therapy.

Q: What is the definition of osseointegration?

Osseointegration is the formation of a direct attachment between an implant and bone, without any intervening soft tissue.

Q: Should preoperative antibiotics be given to patients receiving implants?

Laskin et al[6] noted the benefits of prophylactic antibiotics in a study of 2,973 implants. The study demonstrated that patients who receive preoperative antibiotics have a significantly higher survival rate at each phase of treatment.

A Cochrane review by Esposito et al[7] found some evidence suggesting that 2 g amoxicillin given orally 1 hour preoperatively significantly reduces failures of dental implants placed under ordinary conditions. No significant adverse events were reported. The paper states that although it is not certain that postoperative antibiotics are beneficial or which antibiotics are most effective, it might make sense to prescribe a single dose of 2 g amoxicillin prior to implant placement for prophylactic purposes.

Q: Describe some differences between natural teeth and implants.

- Host response: Schierano et al[8] found no significant differences between implants and teeth in terms of both pro- and anti-inflammatory cytokines. Lang et al[9] reported that while plasma cells and lymphocytes dominated in both types of lesions, neutrophil granulocytes and macrophages occurred in larger proportions in peri-implantitis than in periodontitis. The condition is self-limiting around teeth but not around implants.
- Bacteria: Leonhardt et al[10] found no significant microbiologic difference between titanium implants and teeth in healthy conditions and in gingivitis and periodontitis. According to Lang et al,[9] because a host response is a reaction to a bacterial challenge, there is no reason to assume that it will be different in the peri-implant mucosa when compared with the gingiva.
- Periodontal ligament: Implants do not have a periodontal ligament, but they do have sulcular and junctional epithelia. They have a more limited vascular supply than those of teeth.
- Removal of plaque and calculus: Speelman et al[11] noted that fixed deposits are more easily removed from titanium surfaces than from natural teeth. According to LeBeau,[12] calculus and plaque should be easier to remove from the implant surface than from natural teeth.
- Peri-implant mucositis versus gingivitis: Lang et al[9] found that in the onset of mucositis/gingivitis, there is no evidence that the host response to the bacterial challenge is different at tooth and implant sites. Both mucositis and gingivitis are reversible.

- Conversion of mucositis to peri-implantitis versus that of gingivitis to peri-odontitis: Lang et al[9] assumed, based on data, that mucositis lesions may progress to peri-implantitis earlier than gingivitis converts to periodontitis. The paper also found that the apical extension of the lesion was more pronounced in peri-implantitis than in periodontitis.

Q: What are some of the surface modifications used to create a rough surface of a dental implant?

Surface modifications of implants include[13]:

- Grit-blasted or grit-blasted and acid-etched
- Microgrooved or plasma-sprayed titanium
- Plasma-sprayed hydroxyapatite coatings
- TiUnite (Nobel Biocare) (crystalline and phosphate enriched)

Q: Are rough surface implants more successful than smooth surface implants?

According to Cochran,[3] rough surfaces have a superior success rate for all implants, regardless of location, compared with smooth surfaces (Fig 13-4).

Khang et al[14] found that 36 (12 dual acid-etched and 24 machined surface) implants failed out of 432 implants (247 dual acid-etched, 185 machined surface). The collective success rates were 86.7% for the machined surface implants and 95% for the dual acid-etched implants at 36 months.

Nasatzky et al[15] showed that osteoblasts are sensitive to surface roughness, display-ing decreased proliferation and a more dif-ferentiated phenotype on rougher surfaces. Instead of the usual 12 weeks, roughened titanium implants require a shorter healing period before loading (6 to 8 weeks), which can be advantageous. Shorter (6- to 8-mm) roughened implants can also be employed.

Lang et al[9] found that peri-implantitis is more likely to develop with titanium plasma-sprayed than with minimally rough implants following exposure to the oral environment. Two animal studies further showed that susceptibility to disease progression may be higher for some moderately rough implant surfaces than others.

Fig 13-4 Rough surface implant.

Q: Is keratinized attached tissue around an implant important?

Bouri et al[16] found significantly increased mean Gingival Index and Plaque Index scores, radiographic bone loss, and bleeding on probing for implants with less than 2 mm of keratinized mucosa. They found reduced mean alveolar bone loss and better soft tissue health with greater width of keratinized mucosa around implants.

Chung et al[17] suggested that the lack of adequate keratinized mucosa or attached mucosa around implants, regardless of the surface type, is not associated with increased bone loss.

Q: Are implants placed in patients with periodontal disease successful?

Baelum and Ellegaard[18] found the 5-year survival rate of implants placed in patients with a history of periodontitis to be similar to that observed with implants placed in patients without periodontitis. The authors recommended implant treatment as a good therapeutic option for periodontally compromised patients despite the fact that the 10-year survival rate of one-stage implants was somewhat lower in this population than in individuals without periodontal disease.

Karoussis et al[19] found that a history of chronic periodontitis was associated with significantly greater long-term probing depth, peri-implant marginal bone loss, and peri-implantitis. Ong et al[20] conducted a literature review and found that of the five studies presenting data on implant survival, four reported higher implant survival for non-periodontitis patients in comparison with treated periodontitis patients. The authors also point to evidence of increased implant loss and complications in patients previously treated for periodontitis compared with those with no history of periodontal disease.

Swierkot et al[21] found in their prospective long-term study that patients who were treated for generalized aggressive periodontitis had a 3-fold greater risk of mucositis, a 5-fold greater risk of implant failure, and a 14-fold greater risk of peri-implantitis.

Q: **Where is the greatest force on an implant located?**

The greatest force occurs at the neck of the implant.

Implant Placement

Q: **What presurgical steps need to be taken before implant placement?**

- Restorative requirements, the interarch space and jaw relationships, the location of edentulous areas, and the quantity and quality of available bone should be evaluated before implants are selected as a treatment option. It is also a good idea to get study casts and photographs to be able to perform case analysis when the patient is not present.[13]
- Radiographs and cone beam images are necessary to determine the height of available bone in three dimensions and for selection of the dimensions of the implants. They also may be needed to determine the location of anatomical structures (eg, nerves and vessels).
- Written informed consent must be obtained from the patient.

Q: **Describe the basic technique for implant placement.**

The basic implant placement technique is outlined in Fig 13-5.

After the patient has been anesthetized, a full-thickness incision (a tissue punch can also be used in some cases) is made in keratinized attached tissue in the edentulous area. A vertical incision may be needed for reflection.

A periosteal elevator is used to raise the flap. Great care must be taken to avoid any tears in the flap.

After the bone is exposed, the implants are placed based on manufacturer recommendations (radiographs with direction indicators should be taken to ensure proper angulation).

A cover screw or healing abutment is placed, and the flaps are sutured.

Fig 3-5 Implant placement technique.

Fig 13-6 *(a)* Incision made for implant placement in keratinized attached tissue. *(b)* Direction indicators placed.

There are three principles that must be followed when placing implants[13] (Fig 13-6):

1. The surgical procedure must minimize thermal trauma to the bone. Copious irrigation should be used to avoid overheating of the bone.
2. A primary healing period of variable duration must be allowed to permit osseointegration to be achieved (some studies are starting to question this principle).
3. There should be no micromotion greater than 100 µm during the healing period.

If multiple implants are to be placed, it has been found that arranging implants in a nonlinear manner creates a more stable base that is more resistant to torquing forces.

Q: How much anterior-posterior (A-P) spread is needed in the maxilla and mandible when an implant-supported prosthesis is treatment planned?

A-P spread is the distance from the center of the most anterior implant to the distal surface of the most posterior implant.

- Maxilla: An A-P spread of 2 cm with six implants. The cantilever length should not exceed half the A-P spread.
- Mandible: An A-P spread of 1 cm with four implants. The cantilever length should not exceed twice the A-P spread.

Q: What is the difference between a single-stage technique and a two-stage technique?

- Single-stage: The implant is exposed, and a healing abutment or restoration (most likely provisional) is placed but not loaded.

- Two-stage: The implant is placed and covered with a cover screw and gingiva. After 3 to 6 months, the implant is exposed, and a healing abutment and subsequently the restoration are placed.

Q: How much space is needed between the apex of an implant and the mental nerve?

A minimum of 2 mm is needed between the apex of an implant and the mental nerve.

Implants and Esthetics

Q: What does the distance from the interproximal contact point to the crest of bone have to be to have the papilla present 100% of the time?

Tarnow et al[22] found that the papilla was present 100% of the time when the measurement from the interproximal contact point to the crest of bone was 5 mm or less. The papilla was present 56% of the time when the distance was 6 mm, and the papilla was present 27% of the time or less when the distance was 7 mm or more.

Tarnow et al[23] also found that between two neighboring implants, the average height of papillary tissue was 3.4 mm, with a range of 1 to 7 mm. The most frequently probed heights were 2 mm (16.9%), 3 mm (35.3%), and 4 mm (37.5%).

Q: What does the distance between two implants and between an implant and a tooth have to be to preserve interdental bone?

According to Tarnow et al,[23] the distance between two implants should be at least 3 mm in order to preserve interdental bone (Fig 13-7). Vela et al[24] recommended 1.5 mm between the implant and the tooth to maintain bone adjacent to the teeth and 1 mm between the implant and the tooth when using platform-switched implants.

Fig 13-7 *(a)* Intraoral view before extractions. *(b)* Maxillary implants placed. *(c)* Mandibular implants placed.

Q: What should be evaluated when placing an anterior implant?

The following should be included in the evaluation prior to placing an anterior implant[25]:

- Mesiodistal dimension of the edentulous area
- Three-dimensional radiographs of the site
- Neighboring teeth (tooth dimensions, form, position, and orientation; periodontal/endodontic status; length of roots; crown-to-root ratio)
- Interarch relationships (vertical dimension of occlusion, interocclusal space)
- Esthetic parameters (height of upper smile line, lower lip line, occlusal plane orientation, dental and facial symmetry)
- Patient expectations
- Plaque control
- Primary stability of the implant

Q: What are the contraindications for immediate implant placement in the esthetic zone?

- Heavy smoker
- Patient with very high expectations
- Immunocompromised patient
- Highly scalloped and thin biotype
- Triangular crowns
- Soft tissue defects
- High lip line

Q: What surgical guidelines need to be followed for placement of an esthetic implant?

Figure 13-8 presents the surgical guidelines for placing esthetic implants.

Low-trauma surgical principles	Precise three-dimensional positioning	Slightly palatal positioning to preserve keratinized attached labial tissue

	Use of a screw-retained implant to prevent subgingival cement placement	Deeper placement of the implant to allow the superstructure to be hidden and a gradual emergence profile

Fig 13-8 Surgical guidelines for esthetic implant placement.

Q: **How thick is the buccal wall in the esthetic area?**

Huynh-Ba et al[26] suggested that thin (≤ 1 mm) buccal walls were found in most extraction sites in the anterior maxilla. As a result, augmentation procedures are necessary to attain sufficient bony contours around the implant in most clinical situations.

Q: **Does soft tissue grafting of the maxillary anterior area after immediate implant placement result in a gain of volume?**

Grunder[27] did a study on 24 patients, with 12 in the grafted group (a subepithelial connective tissue graft was placed using the tunnel technique at the time of tooth extraction and implant placement) and 12 in the nongrafted group. Measurements of the labial volume were taken before treatment and 6 months after implant placement. The nongrafted group lost a mean of 1.063 mm of volume, as opposed to the grafted group, which gained 0.34 mm. At the time of immediate implant placement in the esthetic zone, insertion of a soft tissue graft can be advantageous.

Q: **What is the survival rate of a single anterior implant placed immediately after extraction?**

The mean survival rate based on many studies[28] is 97%.

Implant Shape and Length

Q: **When can short implants be used?**

Figure 13-9 presents the indications for placing short implants.

Fig 13-9 Indications for short implants.

Q: Are short implants successful?

Fugazzotto[29] performed retrospective analysis on 1,774 patients and placed 2,073 implants of 6, 7, 8, or 9 mm in length. The implants were either supporting short-span fixed prostheses or single crowns. The survival rates for the implants were 98.1% to 99.7%. The study concluded that survival rates for implants 6 to 9 mm in length are comparable to those of longer implants.

Q: What are the main implant shapes?

Tapered and straight are the main implant shapes (Fig 13-10).

Tapered implants avoid anatomical structures that may be close to the apex of the implant.

Moon et al[30] found that for tapered screw-type implants, underpreparation significantly increased the implant stability quotient (ISQ), whereas overpreparation significantly decreased the ISQ value.

Tapered implants have more surface area.

Screw-type (tapered) vs cylindric (straight)

Fig 13-10 Tapered versus straight implants.

Immediate Implants

Q: When can an immediate implant be useful?

If there is potential for postextraction bone resorption and ridge deformation, an immediate implant can be effective provided that stability is achieved.[13]

However, Araújo et al[31] discovered that implant placement in the extraction site did not stop the remodeling that occurred in the walls of the socket. At 3 months, they found that the buccal and lingual wall heights were similar in implant and edentulous sites.

Q: Can an immediate implant achieve osseointegration?

Wilson et al[32] conducted a histologic study of implants placed in immediate extraction sites and noted that titanium plasma-sprayed implants can achieve osseointegration when placed immediately into extraction sockets. They also found that the most critical aspect relating to the ultimate extent of bone-implant contact is the horizontal component of the peri-implant defect.

If there is a distance of more than 2 mm from the socket to the implant, bone graft materials are required to ensure success. Kahnberg[33] demonstrated a submerged surgical technique that had satisfactory clinical and radiographic outcomes over a 2-year period in 26 patients. The study noted that using autologous bone graft material to fill the gap between implant and labial bone resulted in implants being placed effectively in fresh extraction sockets.

Artzi et al[34] demonstrated that both delayed and immediate placement of implants are clinically effective, but immediate placement of implants leads to greater bone resorption around the implant neck and as a result decreases implant stability.

Q: What is the success rate for immediate implants?

In a prospective clinical trial of 134 implants in 81 patients, Becker et al[35] placed implants at the time of tooth extraction without barrier membranes or graft materials. The cumulative success rate for the 47 implants with 4- to 5-year follow-up was 93.3%.

Al-Shabeeb et al[36] suggested that multiple immediate implants placed in contiguous extraction sites are associated with significantly greater buccal bone remodeling than that seen with single a immediate implant placed in an extraction site.

Covani et al[37] conducted a prospective clinical study that found that immediate implants have a 91.8% success rate after 10 years. Guided bone regeneration made no difference in the success or survival of implants. During the 10-year evaluation, the clinical attachment level, marginal bone loss, and soft tissue measurements were stable.

Platform Switching

Q: What is platform switching?

Platform switching is the use of an abutment that is smaller than the implant. The theory is that the microgap is reduced and there is less bone loss.

Q: Has platform switching been shown to be effective?

Cappiello et al[38] found that the vertical bone loss for patients who did not receive a platform-switched abutment was between 1.3 and 2.1 mm. Patients who received an abutment 1 mm narrower than the platform had vertical bone loss between 0.6 and 1.2 mm. These figures validate the significant role of the microgap between the abutment and the implant in the remodeling of the peri-implant crestal bone. Not only does platform switching increase the long-term predictability of implant therapy, but it also reduces peri-implant crestal bone resorption.

Canullo et al[39] found that the group that received a narrower abutment had a bone reduction level of 0.30 mm, whereas the control had a bone reduction level of 1.19 mm. The study did not find differences between the two groups in bleeding on probing and pocket probing depth.

Effect of Smoking on Implants

Q: What is the failure rate of implants in smokers?

Strietzel et al[40] conducted a meta-analysis and found that smokers had a greater risk of implant failure (implant-related odds ratio [OR] of 2.25) compared with nonsmokers. The OR for implant placement with augmentation was 3.61 in smokers. Overall, the review suggested that the risk of biologic complications is significantly higher for smokers than for nonsmokers.

Moy et al[41] found that smokers had a relative risk ratio of 1.56 for implant failure. They noted that implant failure significantly increased among patients who were 60 years or older, smoked, had a history of diabetes or head and neck radiation, or were postmenopausal and taking hormone replacement therapy.

The reasons behind the high failure rate of implants in smokers include the following[42]:

- Carbon monoxide reduces oxygenation of the healing tissues.
- Nicotine is vasoconstrictive, increasing platelet aggregation and adhesiveness and reducing blood flow.
- Cytotoxic effects on fibroblasts and polymorphonuclear cells disrupt cell repair and defense.
- Wound healing is impaired, leading to a higher complication rate.

Peri-implantitis

Q: What is peri-implantitis?

Peri-implantitis is defined as an inflammatory process affecting the tissue around an implant in function that has resulted in loss of supporting bone. Anaerobic bacteria are the primary factor for bone loss and have been observed in the sulcus of implants, especially when probing depths are greater than 5 mm.[43]

Q: What can cause peri-implantitis?

- Cement trapped below the gingiva
- Inadequate seating of the restoration on the abutment
- Overcontouring the restoration
- Implant malpositioning

In a retrospective study, Quirynen et al[44] noted that endodontic pathology of an extracted tooth (scar tissue–impacted tooth), residual granulomatous tissue at the recipient site, or potential endodontic pathology from a neighboring tooth can trigger retrograde peri-implantitis.

Heitz-Mayfield[45] found substantial evidence that the following was associated with peri-implantitis:

- Poor oral hygiene
- History of periodontitis
- Cigarette smoking

There is limited evidence that the following is associated with peri-implantitis:

- Poorly controlled diabetes
- Alcohol consumption

Berglundh et al[46] proposed that the development of peri-implantitis, if untreated, is less distinct at implants with a polished surface than at implants with a moderately rough surface (sandblasted acid-etched surfaces).

Q: In what percentage of patients do peri-implant mucositis and peri-implantitis occur?

Lindhe et al[47] noted that peri-implantitis occurs in between 28% and 56% of patients treated with implants and peri-implant mucositis occurs in about 80% of patients.

Q: How should peri-implantitis be treated?

Figure 13-11 presents considerations for the treatment of peri-implantitis according to Lindhe et al.[47]

Bacterial deposits must be removed in the treatment of peri-implant mucositis and peri-implantitis.

The clinician should be aware that peri-implantitis is difficult to treat and the outcomes may not be predictable.

If nonsurgical mechanical therapy does not resolve the lesion, adjunctive antimicrobials and access flap surgery are recommended.

In order to restore the hard tissue defect, reconstructive surgery may be considered.

Fig 13-11 Treatment of peri-implantitis.

Byrne[48] noted that the evidence is inconclusive regarding the most effective method of treating peri-implantitis. In most cases, simple mechanical debridement seemed to achieve results that were similar to those of more complex therapies.

Implant Hygiene

Q: What instruments can be used on implant surfaces?

Mengel et al[49] studied the effect of the Densonic sonic scaler (Senova) with universal tips, the Cavitron Jet ultrasonic unit (Dentsply), a plastic curette, a titanium curette, and the Gracey curette on the implant surface. All instruments except the rubber cup and Cavitron Jet air polishing system left marked traces at the transition of the implant head to the titanium plasma coating of the full-screw implants. The study found that the plastic curette, Cavitron Jet air polishing system, Densonic sonic scaler (in some situations), and rubber tip are appropriate for cleaning the implant surface.

Fox et al[50] found that metal instruments considerably changed the titanium surface, as opposed to plastic instruments, which produced an insignificant alteration of the implant surface.

Sinus Elevation

Q: What percent of sinuses have septa?

According to Ulm et al,[51] 30% of sinuses have septa (usually in the middle) between the second premolar and first molar.

Q: **Describe the shape and dimensions of the maxillary sinus.**

The maxillary sinus is pyramidal in shape. It averages 3.75 cm in height and 2.5 cm in width. Its anteroposterior depth averages 3 cm.

Q: **What is the blood supply to the sinus?**

Blood is supplied to the sinus through the posterior superior alveolar artery, infraorbital artery, and posterior superior nasal artery.

Q: **What is the innervation to the sinus?**

The superior alveolar nerves (anterior, medial, and posterior) and infraorbital nerve innervate the sinus.

Q: **Describe how to perform a sinus elevation.**

Boyne and James[52] and Tatum[53] first described the procedure. The lateral window procedure is described in Fig 13-12.

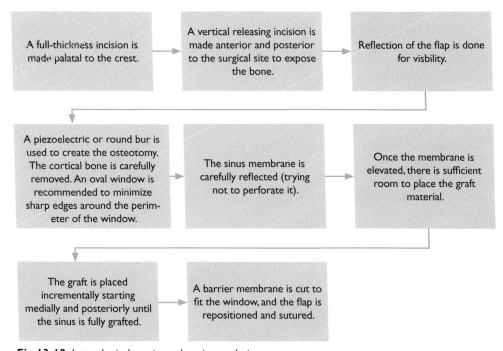

Fig 13-12 Lateral window sinus elevation technique.

Q: What is the average rate of sinus membrane perforation?

Tan et al[54] performed a meta-analysis on the osteotome technique and found that membrane perforation varied between 0% and 21.4%, with a mean of 3.8%.

Malet et al[55] state that perforation of the sinus membrane is the most frequent complication, occurring in about 20% of procedures.

Q: Is there a difference in the rate of sinus membrane perforation when using a round bur versus a piezoelectric instrument?

Wallace et al[56] found that employing the piezoelectric technique reduced the membrane perforation rate (in 100 cases) from the mean reported rate of 30% with rotary instrumentation to 7%. Additionally, all perforations with the piezoelectric technique did not happen with the piezoelectric inserts but during hand instrumentation.

Toscano et al[57] noted that during 56 sinus elevation procedures using the piezoelectric technique, no perforations of the sinus membrane occurred. However, using the hand instrumentation technique, two perforations were noted. The overall sinus perforation rate was 3.6%.

Q: In general, what is the infection rate when a sinus elevation is performed?

Tan et al[54] found that infection was the most common postoperative complication associated with sinus elevation. Of the 19 reviewed studies, with 884 implants, only six reported on postoperative infection. The mean postoperative infection rate was 0.8% (range, 0% to 2.5%).

Malet et al[55] reported an infection rate of grafted sinuses of approximately 3% and graft loss from severe complications at a rate of approximately 2%.

Q: What steps should be taken if a patient develops an infection following a sinus elevation procedure?

Rosen[58] recommends taking the steps presented in Fig 13-13 in cases of postoperative infection following sinus elevation.

Place the patient on a bactericidal antibiotic (eg, amoxicillin).

If the infection is persistent, the site might need to be cultured and a referral made to an otolaryngologist.

If the graft is found to be infected, its removal is necessary.

Fig 13-13 Steps to be taken to treat an infection following sinus elevation.

Q: Which bone material has been found to be the most beneficial for sinus augmentation?

A systematic review by Wallace and Froum[59] found that block grafting of the sinus resulted in a statistically significantly lower implant survival rate (83.3%) than particulate grafts (92.3%). The review found no difference in implant survival between particulate autogenous bone and particulate bone replacement grafts.

Froum et al[60] found anorganic bovine bone to be an effective graft material with 98.2% implant survival.

Piero et al[61] performed a study in which 28 implants were placed in 15 patients (with an average residual bone height of 6.2 mm) with sinus membrane elevation without biomaterials. At the 1-year follow-up, all 28 implants had survived.

Q: Has platelet-rich plasma (PRP) been shown to be beneficial when placed in the sinus?

A review by Wallace and Froum[60] found insufficient data to recommend PRP for sinus graft surgery.

Sánchez et al[62] did not find sufficient dental implant literature regarding the use of PRP. Of the six human studies using PRP, five were case series or reports. The study could not recommend the use of PRP mixed with bone graft material during regeneration procedures due to a lack of scientific evidence. Well-designed, controlled studies are needed to provide evidence for the use of PRP.

Q: What is the success rate of dental implants in a staged sinus elevation procedure?

Bornstein et al[63] found that titanium screw-type implants with a titanium plasma-sprayed or sandblasted, large-grit, acid-etched surface inserted in a two-stage sinus elevation procedure in the posterior maxilla had a 98% 5-year success rate.

Q: Is it necessary to place a membrane over the window?

Tarnow et al[64] studied 12 patients who received sinus elevations with and without placement of a nonresorbable membrane. They found that placement of the barrier membrane tends to increase vital bone formation. It also has a positive effect on implant survival. Those who received a membrane had an implant survival of 100% versus 92.6% for those who did not have a membrane placed.

Tawil and Mawla[65] reported a survival rate of 93.1% for the membrane group and 78.1% for the no-membrane group in their controlled study.

McAllister and Haghighat[66] found that the placement of graft material and a resorbable or nonresorbable barrier membrane over the lateral sinus window aided in graft containment, prevented soft tissue encleftation, and enhanced the implant success rate.

Q: Does the implant surface affect the survival of the implant in the sinus?

Wallace and Froum[59] found that the survival rates of rough surface implants and machined surface implants were 94.6% and 90%, respectively, in the sinus.

Q: Can implants be placed simultaneously with sinus elevation?

The sinus elevation should be performed 4 to 6 months before implant placement if there is 4 to 6 mm of vertical bone between the antral floor and the crest of the ridge. However, if there is greater than 4 to 6 mm of bone, implants can be placed simultaneously as long as they are stable (Fig 13-14).

Fig 13-14 Implant placement and sinus augmentation performed simultaneously.

Osteotome

Q: **What is the osteotome technique?**

Summers[67] introduced the bone-added osteotome sinus floor elevation procedure in 1994. The sinus floor is elevated by inward collapse of the residual crestal floor with specially designed osteotomes. Bone graft material can be introduced through the prepared osteotomy, if needed, with or without simultaneous implant placement. The amount of augmentation achieved by the osteotome technique was 3 to 5 mm.[66]

Q: **What is the minimum bone height needed to perform the osteotome technique?**

Rosen et al[68] treated 101 patients with 174 implants. Screw-type and cylindric implants with machined, titanium plasma-sprayed, and hydroxyapatite surfaces from different manufacturers were used. When pretreatment bone height was 5 mm or more, the survival rate was 96% or higher; however, when pretreatment bone height was 4 mm or less, the survival rate fell to 85.7%. Preexisting bone height between the sinus floor and the crest was the most important factor influencing implant survival.

Toffler[69] found that the osteotome technique has a survival rate of 93.5%. The survival rate fell to 73.3% when only sites with a residual bone height of 4 mm or less were considered. The height of the residual alveolar ridge was the chief determinant. Graft material, implant design, and the method of sinus floor infracture (direct or bone-cushioned) exerted minimal influence on survival outcome; conversely, issues such as an overdenture prosthesis, edentulism, and osteoporosis were shown to negatively impact postloading survival of implants placed in regions of limited residual bone height.

Alternatives to Implants

Q: **Are fixed partial dentures a better option than an implant-supported single implant? How does root canal therapy compare with both options?**

Torabinejad et al[70] found success rates for root canal therapy and fixed partial dentures to be lower than those for an implant-supported single implant, yet success criteria differed greatly among the various treatments, which makes comparisons challenging. A stand-alone implant and root canal therapy had survival rates comparable and superior to that of fixed partial dentures.

Salinas and Eckert[71] performed a systematic review and found that fixed partial dentures of all designs at 60 months exhibited an 84.0% success rate, while single-implant restorations at 60 months demonstrated a 95.1% success rate.

Iqbal and Kim[72] found no substantial dissimilarities in survival between single-tooth implants and restored root canal–treated teeth.

Q: What are the alternatives to implants?

Figure 13-15 presents the alternatives to implant placement.

Implant alternatives
- Fixed partial denture
- Orthodontics to close the space
- Removable partial denture
- No treatment

Fig 13-15 Alternatives to implant placement.

Miscellaneous

Q: Is there a difference in success rate with placement of an implant in a clean versus a sterile condition?

Scharf and Tarnow[73] found implant success rates of 98.9% under sterile conditions and 98.2% under clean conditions (not statistically significant). In order to attain a similar high rate of osseointegration, implant surgery can be performed under both sterile and clean conditions.

Q: Describe the interface between an implant and the epithelium.

The interface between an implant and the epitheilum consists of hemidesmosomes and basal lamina. The biologic width is 3 to 4 mm with 2 mm of epithelial attachment and 1 mm of connective tissue attachment. Collagen fibers are parallel to the implant.

Q: What is the survival rate of implants placed in irradiated bone?

Buddula et al[74] did a retrospective study and found that implants placed in patients with head and neck cancer who had received radiation treatment had a greater risk of failure compared with those placed in nonirradiated bone. The survival of the implants at 1 year was 98.9%, at 5 years 89.9%, and at 10 years 72.3%. The study also found that implants placed in the maxilla had a greater chance of failure than those placed in the mandible. Lastly, implants placed in the posterior region had a greater likelihood of failure than those placed anteriorly.

Q: Can an implant be placed in sclerotic bone?

A cone beam computed tomography scan, preferably with high resolution and a small field of view, should be ordered to assess how sclerotic the bone is and the extent of the changes. The problem with sclerotic bone is the decreased vascularity, which may compromise healing and osseointegration.

References

1. Brånemark PI, Zarb GA, Albrektsson T (eds). Tissue-Integrated Prostheses. Chicago: Quintessence, 1985.
2. Zarb GA, Albrektsson T. Criteria for determining clinical success with osseointegrated dental implants [in French]. Cah Prothese 1990;(71):19–26.
3. Cochran DL. A comparison of endosseous dental implant surfaces. J Periodontol 1999;70:1523–1539.
4. Adell R, Lekholm U, Rockler B, Brånemark PI. A 15-year study of osseointegrated implants in the treatment of the edentulous jaw. Int J Oral Surg 1981;10:387–416.
5. Becker W, Becker BE, Alsuwyed A, Al-Mubarak S. Long-term evaluation of 282 implants in maxillary and mandibular molar positions: A prospective study. J Periodontol 1999;70:896–901.
6. Laskin DM, Dent CD, Morris HF, Ochi S, Olson JW. The influence of preoperative antibiotics on success of endosseous implants at 36 months. Ann Periodontol 2000;5:166–174.
7. Esposito M, Grusovin MG, Loli V, Coulthard P, Worthington HV. Does antibiotic prophylaxis at implant placement decrease early implant failures? A Cochrane systematic review. Eur J Oral Implantol 2010;3:101–110.
8. Schierano G, Pejrone G, Roana J, et al. A split-mouth study on microbiological profile in clinical healthy teeth and implants related to key inflammatory mediators. Int J Immunopathol Pharmacol 2010;23:279–288.
9. Lang NP, Berglundh T; Working Group 4 of Seventh European Workshop on Periodontology. Periimplant diseases: Where are we now?—Consensus of the Seventh European Workshop on Periodontology. J Clin Periodontol 2011;38(suppl 11):178–181.
10. Leonhardt A, Berglundh T, Ericsson I, Dahlén G. Putative periodontal pathogens on titanium implants and teeth in experimental gingivitis and periodontitis in beagle dogs. Clin Oral Implants Res 1992;3:112–119.
11. Speelman JA, Collaert B, Klinge B. Evaluation of different methods to clean titanium abutments. A scanning electron microscopic study. Clin Oral Implants Res 1992;3:120–127.
12. LeBeau J. Maintaining the long-term health of the dental implant and the implant-borne restoration. Compend Contin Educ Oral Hyg 1997;3(3):3–10.

13. The Research, Science and Therapy Committee of the American Academy of Periodontology. Position paper: Dental implants in periodontal therapy. J Periodontol 2000;71:1934–1942.

14. Khang W, Feldman S, Hawley CE, Gunsolley J. A multi-center study comparing dual acid-etched and machined-surfaced implants in various bone qualities. J Periodontol 2001;72:1384–1390.

15. Nasatzky E, Gultchin J, Schwartz Z. The role of surface roughness in promoting osteointegration [in Hebrew]. Refuat Hapeh Vehashinayim 2003;20:8–19,98.

16. Bouri A Jr, Bissada N, Al-Zahrani MS, Faddoul F, Nouneh I. Width of keratinized gingiva and the health status of the supporting tissues around dental implants. Int J Oral Maxillofac Implants 2008;23:323–326.

17. Chung DM, Oh TJ, Shotwell JL, Misch CE, Wang HL. Significance of keratinized mucosa in maintenance of dental implants with different surfaces. J Periodontol 2006;77:1410–1420.

18. Baelum V, Ellegaard B. Implant survival in periodontally compromised patients. J Periodontol 2004;75:1404–1412.

19. Karoussis IK, Kotsovilis S, Fourmousis I. A comprehensive and critical review of dental implant prognosis in periodontally compromised partially edentulous patients. Clin Oral Implants Res 2007;18:669–679.

20. Ong CT, Ivanovski S, Needleman IG, et al. Systematic review of implant outcomes in treated periodontitis subjects. J Clin Periodontol 2008;35:438–462.

21. Swierkot K, Lottholz P, Flores-de-Jacoby L, Mengel R. Mucositis, peri-implantitis, implant success, and survival of implants in patients with treated generalized aggressive periodontitis: 3- to 16-year results of a prospective long-term cohort study. J Periodontol 2012;83:1213–1225.

22. Tarnow DP, Magner AW, Fletcher P. The effect of the distance from the contact point to the crest of bone on the presence or absence of the interproximal dental papilla. J Periodontol 1992;63:995–996.

23. Tarnow D, Elian N, Fletcher P, et al. Vertical distance from the crest of bone to the height of the interproximal papilla between adjacent implants. J Periodontol 2003;74:1785–1788.

24. Vela X, Méndez V, Rodríguez X, Segalá M, Tarnow DP. Crestal bone changes on platform-switched implants and adjacent teeth when the tooth-implant distance is less than 1.5 mm. Int J Periodontics Restorative Dent 2012;32:149–155.

25. Besler U, Vernard JP, Buser D. Implant placement in the esthetic zone: In: Lindhe J, Karring T, Lang NP (eds). Clinical Periodontology and Implant Dentistry, ed 4. Oxford, UK: Blackwell Munksgaard, 2003:918.

26. Huynh-Ba G, Pjetursson BE, Sanz M, et al. Analysis of the socket bone wall dimensions in the upper maxilla in relation to immediate implant placement. Clin Oral Implants Res 2010;21:37–42.

27. Grunder U. Crestal ridge width changes when placing implants at the time of tooth extraction with and without soft tissue augmentation after a healing period of 6 months: Report of 24 consecutive cases. Int J Periodontics Restorative Dent 2011;31:9–17.

28. Wöhrle PS. Single-tooth replacement in the aesthetic zone with immediate provisionalization: Fourteen consecutive case reports. Pract Periodontics Aesthet Dent 1998;10:1107–1114.

29. Fugazzotto PA. Shorter implants in clinical practice: rationale and treatment results. Int J Oral Maxillofac Implants 2008;23:487–496.

30. Moon SH, Um HS, Lee JK, Chang BS, Lee MK. The effect of implant shape and bone preparation on primary stability. J Periodontal Implant Sci 2010;40:239–243.

31. Araújo MG, Sukekava F, Wennström JL, Lindhe J. Ridge alterations following implant placement in fresh extraction sockets: An experimental study in the dog. J Clin Periodontol 2005;32:645–652.

32. Wilson TG Jr, Schenk R, Buser D, Cochran D. Implants placed in immediate extraction sites: a report of histologic and histometric analyses of human biopsies. Int J Oral Maxillofac Implants 1998;13:333–341.

33. Kahnberg KE. Immediate implant placement in fresh extraction sockets: A clinical report. Int J Oral Maxillofac Implants 2009;24:282–288.

34. Artzi Z, Nemcovsky CE, Tal H, Kozlovsky A. Timing of implant placement and augmentation with bone replacement material: Clinical assessment at 8 and 16 months [epub ahead of print 2011 Dec 16]. Clin Implant Dent Relat Res doi: 10.1111/j.1708-8208.2011.00421.x.

35. Becker BE, Becker W, Ricci A, Geurs N. A prospective clinical trial of endosseous screw-shaped implants placed at the time of tooth extraction without augmentation. J Periodontol 1998;69:920–926.

36. Al-Shabeeb MS, Al-Askar M, Al-Rasheed A, et al. Alveolar bone remodeling around immediate implants placed in accordance with the extraction socket classification: A three-dimensional microcomputed tomography analysis. J Periodontol 2012;83:981–987.

37. Covani U, Chiappe G, Bosco M, Orlando B, Quaranta A, Barone A. A 10-year evaluation of implants placed in fresh extraction sockets: A prospective cohort study. J Periodontol 2012;83:1226–1234.

38. Cappiello M, Luongo R, Di Iorio D, Bugea C, Cocchetto R, Celletti R. Evaluation of peri-implant bone loss around platform-switched implants. Int J Periodontics Restorative Dent 2008;28:347–355.

39. Canullo L, Goglia G, Iurlaro G, Iannello G. Short-term bone level observations associated with platform switching in immediately placed and restored single maxillary implants: a preliminary report. Int J Prosthodont 2009;22:277–282.

40. Strietzel FP, Reichart PA, Kale A, Kulkarni M, Wegner B, Küchler I. Smoking interferes with the prognosis of dental implant treatment: A systematic review and meta-analysis. J Clin Periodontol 2007;34:523–544.

41. Moy PK, Medina D, Shetty V, Aghaloo TL. Dental implant failure rates and associated risk factors. Int J Oral Maxillofac Implants 2005;20:569–577.

42. Liddelow G, Klineberg I. Patient-related risk factors for implant therapy. A critique of pertinent literature. Aust Dent J 2011;56:417–426.

43. Misch CE, Perel ML, Wang HL, et al. Implant success, survival, and failure: The International Congress of Oral Implantologists (ICOI) Pisa Consensus Conference. Implant Dent 2008;17:5–15.

44. Quirynen M, Vogels R, Alsaadi G, Naert I, Jacobs R, van Steenberghe D. Predisposing conditions for retrograde peri-implantitis, and treatment suggestions. Clin Oral Implants Res 2005;16:599–608.

45. Heitz-Mayfield LJ. Peri-implant diseases: Diagnosis and risk indicators. J Clin Periodontol 2008;35(8 suppl):292–304.

46. Berglundh T, Gotfredsen K, Zitzmann NU, Lang NP, Lindhe J. Spontaneous progression of ligature induced peri-implantitis at implants with different surface roughness: An experimental study in dogs. Clin Oral Implants Res 2007;18:655–661.

47. Lindhe J, Meyle J; Group D of European Workshop on Periodontology. Peri-implant diseases: Consensus Report of the Sixth European Workshop on Periodontology. J Clin Periodontol 2008;35(8 suppl):282–285.

48. Byrne G. Effectiveness of different treatment regimens for peri-implantitis. J Am Dent Assoc 2012;143:391–392.

49. Mengel R, Buns CE, Mengel C, Flores-de-Jacoby L. An in vitro study of the treatment of implant surfaces with different instruments. Int J Oral Maxillofac Implants 1998;13:91–96.

50. Fox SC, Moriarty JD, Kusy RP. The effects of scaling a titanium implant surface with metal and plastic instruments: An in vitro study. J Periodontol 1990;61:485–490.

51. Ulm CW, Solar P, Krennmair G, Matejka M, Watzek G. Incidence and suggested surgical management of septa in sinus-lift procedures. Int J Oral Maxillofac Implants 1995;10:462–465.

52. Boyne PJ, James RA. Grafting of the maxillary sinus floor with autogenous marrow and bone. J Oral Surg 1980;38:613–616.

53. Tatum H Jr. Maxillary and sinus implant reconstructions. Dent Clin North Am 1986;30:207–229.

54. Tan WC, Lang NP, Zwahlen M, Pjetursson BE. A systematic review of the success of sinus floor elevation and survival of implants inserted in combination with sinus floor elevation. Part II: Transalveolar technique. J Clin Periodontol 2008;35(8 suppl):241–254.

55. Malet J, Mora F, Bouchard P. Implant Dentistry at-a-Glance. Chichester, West Sussex, UK: Wiley-Blackwell, 2012:89.

56. Wallace SS, Mazor Z, Froum SJ, Cho SC, Tarnow DP. Schneiderian membrane perforation rate during sinus elevation using piezosurgery: Clinical results of 100 consecutive cases. Int J Periodontics Restorative Dent 2007;27:413–419.

57. Toscano NJ, Holtzclaw D, Rosen PS. The effect of piezoelectric use on open sinus lift perforation: A retrospective evaluation of 56 consecutively treated cases from private practices. J Periodontol 2010;81:167–171.

58. Rosen PS. Complications with the bone-added osteotome sinus floor elevation: Etiology, prevention, and treatment. In: Froum S (ed). Dental Implant Complications: Etiology, Prevention, and Treatment. Oxford, UK: Blackwell Publishing, 2010:310–324.

59. Wallace SS, Froum SJ. Effect of maxillary sinus augmentation on the survival of endosseous dental implants. A systematic review. Ann Periodontol 2003;8:328–343.

60. Froum SJ, Tarnow DP, Wallace SS, Rohrer MD, Cho SC. Sinus floor elevation using anorganic bovine bone matrix (OsteoGraf/N) with and without autogenous bone: A clinical, histologic, radiographic, and histomorphometric analysis—Part 2 of an ongoing prospective study. Int J Periodontics Restorative Dent 1998;18:528–543.

61. Piero B, Mario V, Niccolò N, Marco F. Implant placement in combination with sinus membrane elevation without biomaterials: A 1-year study on 15 patients. Clin Implant Dent Relat Res 2012;14:682–689.

62. Sánchez AR, Sheridan PJ, Kupp LI. Is platelet-rich plasma the perfect enhancement factor? A current review. Int J Oral Maxillofac Implants 2003;18:93–103.

63. Bornstein MM, Chappuis V, Von Arx T, Buser D. Performance of dental implants after staged sinus floor elevation procedures: 5-year results of a prospective study in partially edentulous patients. Clin Oral Implants Res 2008;19:1034–1043.

64. Tarnow DP, Wallace SS, Froum SJ, Rohrer MD, Cho SC. Histologic and clinical comparison of bilateral sinus floor elevations with and without barrier membrane placement in 12 patients: Part 3 of an ongoing prospective study. Int J Periodontics Restorative Dent 2000;20:117–125.

65. Tawil G, Mawla M. Sinus floor elevation using a bovine bone mineral (Bio-Oss) with or without the concomitant use of a bilayered collagen barrier (Bio-Gide): A clinical report of immediate and delayed implant placement. Int J Oral Maxillofac Implants 2001;16:713–721.

66. McAllister BS, Haghighat K. Bone augmentation techniques. J Periodontol 2007;78:377–396.

67. Summers RB. A new concept in maxillary implant surgery: The osteotome technique. Compendium 1994;15:152,154–156,158.

68. Rosen PS, Summers R, Mellado JR, et al. The bone-added osteotome sinus floor elevation technique: Multicenter retrospective report of consecutively treated patients. Int J Oral Maxillofac Implants 1999;14:853–858.

69. Toffler M. Osteotome-mediated sinus floor elevation: A clinical report. Int J Oral Maxillofac Implants 2004;19:266–273.

70. Torabinejad M, Anderson P, Bader J, et al. Outcomes of root canal treatment and restoration, implant-supported single crowns, fixed partial dentures, and extraction without replacement: A systematic review. J Prosthet Dent 2007;98:285–311.

71. Salinas TJ, Eckert SE. In patients requiring single-tooth replacement, what are the outcomes of implant- as compared to tooth-supported restorations? Int J Oral Maxillofac Implants 2007;22(suppl):71–95.

72. Iqbal MK, Kim S. For teeth requiring endodontic treatment, what are the differences in outcomes of restored endodontically treated teeth compared to implant-supported restorations? Int J Oral Maxillofac Implants 2007;22(suppl):96–116.

73. Scharf DR, Tarnow DP. Success rates of osseointegration for implants placed under sterile versus clean conditions. J Periodontol 1993;64:954–956.

74. Buddula A, Assad DA, Salinas TJ, Garces YI, Volz JE, Weaver AL. Survival of dental implants in irradiated head and neck cancer patients: A retrospective analysis. Clin Implant Dent Relat Res 2012;14:716–722.

Inflammation

Background

Q: What are the signs of inflammation?

Rubor (redness), tumor (swelling), calor (heat), dolor (pain), and loss of function are the signs of inflammation.

Q: What is the difference between the innate and the adaptive immune response?

Figure 14-1 presents the characteristics of the innate and adaptive immune responses.

Innate immune response

- Immediate protection through immune cells (macrophages, polymorphonuclear leukocytes [PMNs])
- Not antigen specific

Adaptive immune response

- Recognition of the pathogens (immunologic memory) and a stronger but longer response time through immune cells (B cells and T cells)
- Antigen specific

Fig 14-1 Characteristics of the innate and adaptive immune responses.

Q: Describe the following terms: epigenetics, resolvins, and protectins.

- *Epigenetics:* The relationships between environmental settings and the genetic background to produce a given phenotypical outcome.[1] Includes all meiotically and mitotically inherited changes in gene expression that are not encoded in the DNA sequence itself (DNA methylation or posttranslational modification of histone proteins). According to Martinez et al,[1] dietary and environmental factors in the mother may enhance or reduce epigenetic mechanisms, which may be transmitted intergenerationally or transiently and could be involved in the offspring's susceptibility to obesity and inflammation.
- *Resolvins* and *protectins:* Control the duration and magnitude of inflammation. They are synthesized by omega-3 fatty acids and can stop neutrophil infiltration and chemotaxis. Resolvins (a term derived from *resolution phase interaction products*) have potent anti-inflammatory and immunoregulatory actions, including neutrophil trafficking reduction, cytokine and reactive oxygen species regulation, and inflammatory response decrease. Protectin and neuroprotectin are 10R,17S-dihydroxy docosatrienes, so named given their general anti-inflammatory and protective effects in neural systems, stroke, animal models of Alzheimer disease, and peritonitis.[2]

Q: Describe the five major classes of immunoglobulin (Ig).

IgA
- Important in mucosal immunity
- Found in tears and saliva
- Activates the alternative pathway

IgD
- Found on B lymphocytes
- Usually found with IgM

IgE
- Elicits an immune response by binding to Fc receptors found on the surface of mast cells and basophils and are also found on eosinophils, monocytes, macrophages, and platelets in humans
- Involved in allergies

IgG
- Antibodies are involved in the secondary immune response
- Presence corresponds to maturation of the antibody response
- Can pass through the human placenta, thereby providing protection to the fetus in utero
- Involved in the classic pathway

IgM
- Largest antibody; produced by B cells
- Appears early in infection
- Involved in the classic pathway

Pro-inflammatory Molecules

Q: Which molecules have been associated with bone loss in periodontal disease?

Interleukin-1 (IL-1) and tumor necrosis factor α (TNF-α) are the molecules associated with periodontal disease primarily.[3] Antigen-stimulated lymphocytes (B cells and T cells) also seem to be important. The cascade of events is illustrated in Fig 14-2.

| Antigen-stimulated lymphocytes (B cells and T cells) |

↓

| Receptor activation of nuclear factor-κ B (RANK)–RANK ligand (RANKL)–osteoprotegerin (OPG) axis |

↓

| Increase in the RANKL-OPG ratio and protein production |

↓

| Macrophages are stimulated to osteoclasts and maturation of the osteoclasts |

↓

| Bone loss |

Fig 14-2 Cascade of events leading to bone loss.

Q: Describe the pro-inflammatory molecules.

- IL-1: Both IL-1α and IL-1β are produced by macrophages, monocytes, fibroblasts, and dendritic cells. They form an important part of the inflammatory response of the body against infection. They can promote bone resorption.
- IL-2: Produced by CD4 cells and part of the body's natural response to microbial infection.
- IL-4: Involved in differentiation of CD4[+] T cells into T-helper type 2 (Th2) cells.
- IL-6: Secreted by T cells and macrophages to stimulate the immune response. It can stimulate osteoclasts and plasma cells.

199

- IL-8: Primary function is the induction of chemotaxis in its target cells. It serves as a chemical signal that attracts neutrophils at the site of inflammation.
- IL-10: Anti-inflammatory cytokine.
- C-reactive protein (CRP): Rapid, marked increases in CRP occur with inflammation, infection, trauma and tissue necrosis, malignancies, and autoimmune disorders. An elevated CRP level can provide support for the presence of an inflammatory disease. CRP levels are elevated in patients with periodontitis and may decrease after periodontal therapy.[4]
- Prostaglandin E_2 (PGE$_2$): Stimulates osteoblasts to release factors that stimulate bone resorption by osteoclasts and matrix metalloproteinase (MMP) secretion. Elevated levels of prostaglandins such as PGE$_2$ in inflamed gingiva play a significant role in the tissue destruction caused by periodontitis, in part by targeting local fibroblasts.[5]
- Bradykinin: Increases vascular permeability.
- Interferon-γ (IFN-γ): IFN-γ released by Th1 cells recruits leukocytes to a site of infection, resulting in increased inflammation.
- TNF family: A group of cytokines that can cause cell death (apoptosis).
- Transforming growth factor β (TGF-β): TGF-β1 is the most potent chemoattractant described for human peripheral blood neutrophils (PMNs), suggesting that TGF-β may play a role in the recruitment of PMNs during the initial phase of the inflammatory response.[6]
- MMPs: The collagenases are capable of degrading collagens into distinctive ¾- and ¼-length fragments. These collagens are the major components of bone, cartilage, and dentin.

Q: Which pro-inflammatory molecules have shown an association with diabetes?

Pradhan et al[7] found that elevated levels of CRP and IL-6 can predict the development of type 2 diabetes.

Q: Describe the interaction of CD4 cells with other molecules.

Table 14-1 presents the interaction of CD4 cells (T-helper cells) with other molecules.

Table 14-1 Interaction of CD4 cells with other molecules

	Th1 cell	Th2 cell
Partner	Macrophage	B cell
Cytokine	IL-1β, PGE$_2$, IL-8, and IFN-γ	IL-10, IFN-4, IFN-5, and IFN-6

Q: Can inhibition of IL-1 and TNF reduce the progression of periodontal disease?

Yes, it can. Clinical, radiographic, and biochemical findings by Deo and Bhongade[8] showed in animal models that antagonists to IL-1 and TNF-α block inflammatory cell infiltrate advancement toward the alveolar crest as well as the recruitment of osteoclasts.

Q: Can inhibition of the host response contribute to periodontal tissue destruction?

Yes, neutrophil depletion contributes to periodontal destruction.

Periodontal Disease and Inflammation

Q: Describe the stages from an initial to an advanced lesion.

Figure 14-3 presents the stages from an initial to an advanced lesion.[9]

Initial lesion	Early gingival lesion	Established lesion	Advanced lesion
• After 2 to 4 days of plaque accumulation, inflammation develops. • Neutrophils and macrophages develop. • Although the cellular response develops in 2 to 4 days, the gingiva looks healthy.	• Occurs after 1 week with greater inflammation. • Predominatly see lymphocytes and neutrophils. • Rete peg proliferation and some coronal epithelium is gone. • There is vascular proliferation. • May not shift to gingivitis.	• Occurs at 14 to 21 days. • 10% to 30% plasma cells. • Extravascular IgG is present. • Rete pegs distribute to the connective tissue. • Pocket epithelium is leaky because the junctional epithelium is now pocket epithelium.	• Plaque further extends into the pocket. • Plasma cells predominate. • Loss of connective tissue and alveolar bone. • True periodontal pocket develops. • Irreversible clinical attachment loss.

Fig 14-3 Stages from an initial to an advanced lesion.

Q: What are the theories for periodontal disease progression?

- The continuous model: Most common forms of destructive periodontal disease have been thought to slowly and continuously progress until treatment is provided or tooth loss occurs.
- Random burst or recurrent acute episodes: Rates of attachment loss in individual sites are faster than those consistent with the continuous disease hypothesis or slower than those expected from estimates of prior loss rates. Bursts of activity occur for short periods of time in individual sites.[10]

Q: Describe the inflammatory process of periodontitis.

The inflammatory process of periodontitis is presented in Fig 14-4.

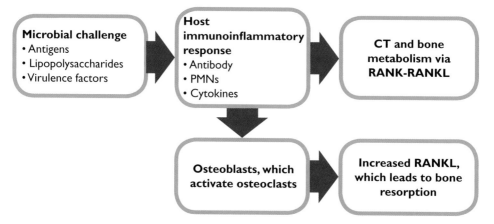

Fig 14-4 Inflammatory process of periodontitis.

Q: How does caloric restriction affect periodontitis?

Reynolds et al[11] found significantly fewer periodontal pockets, a reduced IgG antibody response, and lower IL-8 and ss-glucuronidase levels in male patients who had caloric restriction.

Branch-Mays et al[12] found that caloric restriction has anti-inflammatory effects. The study also suggested that caloric restriction decreases the inflammatory response and reduces active periodontal breakdown associated with an acute microbial challenge.

Abnormalities Associated with Chronic Inflammation

Q: **Describe metabolic disorders and their relationship with inflammation.**

Metabolic disorders are abnormalities that include obesity, high blood pressure, high blood glucose, dyslipidemia, and cardiovascular disease. At the heart of these abnormalities is a pro-inflammatory state.

Obesity, insulin resistance, and type 2 diabetes are closely associated with chronic inflammation characterized by abnormal cytokine production, increased acute-phase reactants and other mediators, and activation of a network of inflammatory signaling pathways.[13] The finding that TNF is overexpressed in the fat cells of obese mice provided the first clear link between obesity, diabetes, and chronic inflammation.[14]

Q: **Describe the relationship between diabetes and inflammation.**

Figures 14-5 and 14-6 present two depictions of the relationship between inflammation and diabetes.

Fig 14-5 Inflammation leading to insulin resistance.

Fig 14-6 Advanced glycation end product (AGE) leading to the release of cytokines and inflammation.

Advanced glycation end product can also prevent development of macrophages involved in repair and thereby delay wound healing. It has also been shown that obesity can increase inflammatory mediators and increase insulin resistance.[15]

Q: What is the relationship between Alzheimer disease (AD) and inflammation?

A recently accepted hallmark of evidence supports the hypothesis of inflammatory processes as viable mechanisms of the pathogenesis of AD. Cojocaru et al[16] found that patients with AD had increased production of the IL-6 cytokine, which indicates that an abnormal cellular immunity may be present. IL-6, which is involved in the pathogenesis of AD, may account for the serum acute-phase proteins found in patients with AD.

Q: Describe the relationship between arthritis and inflammation.

Osteoarthritis (OA) is a multifactorial disorder in which obesity is one of the most influential but modifiable risk factors. Although it has been postulated that obesity is a risk factor simply because it increases mechanical stress on the joints, OA is also prevalent in non-weightbearing areas, such as finger joints, in obese individuals, suggesting another link between obesity and OA—inflammation. Adipose tissues and the infrapatellar fat pad contain cytokines, chemokines, and adipokines (or adipocytokines), which have been shown to have catabolic and pro-inflammatory properties and to coordinate the pathophysiologic processes involved in OA.[17]

Mangge et al[18] found an association between juvenile rheumatoid arthritis and consistent significant fluctuations in serum levels of inflammatory cytokines and soluble receptors.

Miscellaneous

Q: Describe the major histocompatibility complex (MHC) proteins.

- Class I MHC proteins: Found on virtually all cell types and are responsible for presenting fragments of proteins that are synthesized inside the cell. The peptide antigens presented in this manner are checked by killer T cells, which have receptors for the class I MHC proteins. The purpose of this surveillance system is to identify abnormal body cells, such as those infected with viruses or those that have turned malignant.

- Class II MHC proteins: Found only on immune cells such as phagocytes that engulf foreign particles such as bacteria. These cells are specially designed to present peptide antigens derived from such digested particles. The antigens are presented to helper T cells, which have receptors for class II MHC proteins. The purpose of this surveillance system is to stop the immune system from running out of control and attacking the body's own cells.

References

1. Martínez JA, Cordero P, Campión J, Milagro FI. Interplay of early-life nutritional programming on obesity, inflammation and epigenetic outcomes. Proc Nutr Soc 2012;71:276–283.
2. Ariel A, Serhan CN. Resolvins and protectins in the termination program of acute inflammation. Trends Immunol 2007;28:176–183.
3. Cochran DL. Inflammation and bone loss in periodontal disease. J Periodontol 2008;79(8 suppl):1569–1576.
4. Dasanayake AP. C-reactive protein levels are elevated in patients with periodontitis and their CRP levels may go down after periodontal therapy. J Evid Based Dent Pract 2009;9:21–22.
5. Weinberg E, Zeldich E, Weinreb MM, Moses O, Nemcovsky C, Weinreb M. Prostaglandin E$_2$ inhibits the proliferation of human gingival fibroblasts via the EP$_2$ receptor and Epac. J Cell Biochem 2009;108:207–215.
6. Parekh T, Saxena B, Reibman J, Cronstein BN, Gold LI. Neutrophil chemotaxis in response to TGF-beta isoforms (TGF-beta 1, TGF-beta 2, TGF-beta 3) is mediated by fibronectin. J Immunol 1994;152:2456–2466.
7. Pradhan AD, Manson JE, Rifai N, Buring JE, Ridker PM. C-reactive protein, interleukin 6, and risk of developing type 2 diabetes mellitus. JAMA 2001;286:327–334.
8. Deo V, Bhongade ML. Pathogenesis of periodontitis: Role of cytokines in host response. Dent Today 2010;29(9):60–62,64–66.
9. Page RC, Schroeder HE. Pathogenesis of inflammatory periodontal disease. A summary of current work. Lab Invest 1976;34:235–249.
10. Socransky SS, Haffajee AD, Goodson JM, Lindhe J. New concepts of destructive periodontal disease. J Clin Periodontol 1984;11:21–32.
11. Reynolds MA, Dawson DR, Novak KF, et al. Effects of caloric restriction on inflammatory periodontal disease. Nutrition 2009;25:88–97.
12. Branch-Mays GL, Dawson DR, Gunsolley JC, et al. The effects of a calorie-reduced diet on periodontal inflammation and disease in a non-human primate model. J Periodontol 2008;79:1184–1191.
13. Wellen KE, Hotamisligil GS. Inflammation, stress, and diabetes. J Clin Invest 2005;115:1111–1119.
14. Hotamisligil GS, Shargill NS, Spiegelman BM. Adipose expression of tumor necrosis factor-alpha: Direct role in obesity-linked insulin resistance. Science 1993;259(5091):87–91.
15. Cohen DH, Leroith D. Obesity, type 2 diabetes, and cancer: The insulin and IGF connection. Endocr Relat Cancer 2012;19(5):F27–F45.
16. Cojocaru IM, Cojocaru M, Miu G, Sapira V. Study of interleukin-6 production in Alzheimer's disease. Rom J Intern Med 2011;49:55–58.
17. Rai MF, Sandell LJ. Inflammatory mediators: Tracing links between obesity and osteoarthritis. Crit Rev Eukaryot Gene Expr 2011;21:131–142.
18. Mangge H, Kenzian H, Gallistl S, et al. Serum cytokines in juvenile rheumatoid arthritis. Correlation with conventional inflammation parameters and clinical subtypes. Arthritis Rheum 1995;38:211–220.

Oral Medicine

Laboratory Work

Q: What are some important laboratory values?

- Platelet count: 150,000 to 400,000 is normal
- Bleeding time: 2.5 to 8 min is normal
- High-density lipoprotein (HDL): > 50 mg/dL is normal
- Low-density lipoprotein (LDL): < 100 mg/dL is normal
- International normalized ratio (INR): 1 to 1.5 is normal
  - Can treat an INR < 3.5
- Fasting blood sugar:
  - 75 to 100 mg/dL is normal
  - > 126 mg/dL indicates diabetes
  - < 72 mg/dL indicates hypoglycemia
- Hemoglobin A_{1c}: 4% to 6% is normal
  - Can treat patients < 7%
- Body mass index:
  - > 25 kg/m^3 indicates overweight
  - > 30 kg/m^3 indicates obese
- White blood cell count: 4×10^9 to 1.1×10^{10} per liter of blood is normal
- Red blood cell count: 4×10^6 to 6×10^6 is normal
- CD4 counts: 500×10^6 to $1,200 \times 10^6$ is normal
- Neutropenia in adults: count of 1,700 or fewer neutrophils per microliter of blood

- Hemoglobin levels:
  - Adult men: 14 to 18 g/dL is normal
  - Adult women: 12 to 16 g/dL is normal

Q: **What is the normal heart rate?**

- Normal heart rate: 60 to 110 beats per minute (bpm)[1]
- Bradycardia: Less than 60 bpm
- Tachycardia: Greater than 110 bpm

Blood Pressure

Q: **What is the difference between primary and secondary hypertension?**

- Primary hypertension: Most patients (90% to 95%) have primary hypertension. It is idiopathic.
- Secondary hypertension: It may be caused by kidney disease, primary hyperaldosteronism, and pheochromocytoma.

Q: **What are the values for normal blood pressure, prehypertension, and stage 1 and 2 hypertension?**

- Normal blood pressure: 120/80
- Prehypertension: 120 to 139/80 to 89
- Stage 1 hypertension: 140 to 159/90 to 99
- Stage 2 hypertension: 160/100

Q: **What is the classification of blood pressure according to the American Society of Anesthesiologists (ASA)?**

- ASA 1: < 140/< 90
- ASA 2: 140 to 159/90 to 94
- ASA 3: 160 to 199/95 to 114
- ASA 4: > 200/> 115

Q: **Does it make a difference on which arm blood pressure is taken?**

The arm on which blood pressure is measured only makes a difference if the patient has aortic stenosis or a mastectomy.

Q: Are electronic devices as accurate as manual ones in determining the blood pressure of a patient?

Electronic devices are usually accurate to within 3% of a manual sphygmo-manometer.[2]

Q: What can cause errors in blood pressure measurements?

The following factors may cause errors in blood pressure measurements:

• Stress
• Blood pressure may decrease following a big meal
• Caffeine may increase blood pressure

Q: What are the concerns regarding hypertension?

Hypertension can lead to heart disease, stroke, kidney failure, and heart attack.

Q: Describe how hypertension can lead to thrombosis.

Figure 15-1 presents the process by which hypertension can lead to thrombosis.

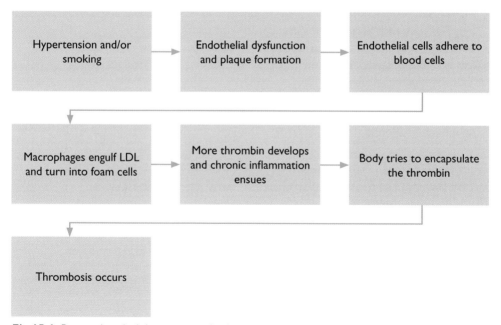

Fig 15-1 Process by which hypertension leads to thrombosis.

Cardiovascular Disease

Q: What are risk factors for cardiovascular disease?

- Patient more than 65 years old
- Smoking
- Systemic blood pressure greater than 140 and diastolic blood pressure greater than 90
- LDL greater than 160
- HDL less than 40
- Fasting blood glucose greater than 120
- Periodontal disease
- Genetics
- Obesity

Q: What does the evidence show about the relationship between cardiovascular disease and periodontal disease?

- A review by Humphrey et al[3] reported on several studies that revealed an independent association of periodontal disease with increased risk for coronary heart disease (CHD). Summary relative risk estimates ranged from 1.24 to 1.34 for different types of periodontal disease (including periodontitis, tooth loss, gingivitis, and bone loss).
- In a meta-analysis of five prospective cohort studies (including 86,092 patients), Bahekar et al[4] found a 1.14-fold increase in risk of developing CHD in individuals with periodontitis compared with controls.
- Beck et al[5] concluded that periodontitis could be considered a risk factor for atherosclerosis/CHD based on the study's finding of an incidence odds ratio of approximately 2.0.
- In a study on 9,760 individuals, DeStefano et al[6] found that those with periodontitis had a 25% increased risk of CHD compared with those who had minimal periodontal disease.

Q: What are the four main theories about the relationship between cardiovascular disease and periodontitis?

1. Direct invasion: Several groups have identified specific oral pathogens in atheromatous tissue.
2. Immunologic sounding: Cytokines and chemokines play a role in activation of endothelium and monocytes associated with developing atheroma[7] (Fig 15-2).
3. Pathogen trafficking: Trafficking of pathogens from the local site of infection to the developing atheroma via inflammatory cells.
4. Autoimmune response: Stimulation of an autoimmune response via molecular mimicry.

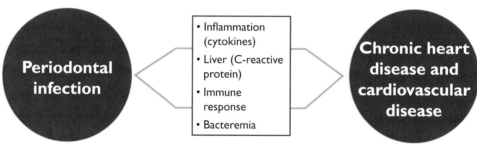

Fig 15-2 Immunologic sounding.

Q: **What are the recommendations for patients who have cardiovascular or periodontal disease?**

Following are the recommendations for patients with cardiovascular or periodontal disease[8]:

- Patients with moderate to severe periodontitis: Patients should be informed that there may be an increased risk for atherosclerotic cardiovascular disease associated with periodontitis.
- Patients with moderate to severe periodontitis who have one known major atherosclerotic cardiovascular disease risk factor (including smoking, immediate family history of cardiovascular disease, or history of dyslipidemia): These patients should consider a medical evaluation if they have not had one in the past 12 months.
- Patients with periodontitis who have two known major atherosclerotic cardiovascular disease risk factors: These patients should be referred for medical evaluation if they have not had one in the past 12 months.

Q: **What are the symptoms of congestive heart failure?**

Fatigue, limited activity, edema, and shortness of breath are symptoms of congestive heart failure. It is important to be aware of orthostatic hypotension with these patients.

Q: **What is the difference between congestive heart failure and a heart attack?**

- Congestive heart failure: The pump and cardiac muscles do not work properly.
- Heart attack/myocardial infarction (MI): There is death of the tissue due to lack of oxygen. There is an interruption of blood supply.

Diabetes

Q: Describe the two types of diabetes.

Defining characteristics of the two types of diabetes are described in Fig 15-3.

Type 1 diabetes	Type 2 diabetes
• Formerly called *insulin-dependent diabetes mellitus*	• Formerly called *non–insulin-dependent diabetes*
• 5% to 10% of diabetic cases; first discovered when patients are young	• 90% to 95% of diabetic patients; discovered midlife and in obese patients
• Immune-mediated destruction of the pancreatic β cells that secrete insulin	• Insulin resistance

Fig 15-3 Defining characteristics of type 1 and type 2 diabetes.

Q: What does hemoglobin A$_{1c}$ measure?

Glycosylate hemoglobin measures the amount of glucose bound to hemoglobin in the red blood cell. Hemoglobin A$_{1c}$ values of 4% to 6% are normal. Patients can be treated with a value of 7% or less. This laboratory result indicates diabetic control over the last 3 months.

Q: What are the possible oral manifestations of diabetes?

The possible oral manifestations of diabetes are shown in Fig 15-4.

Fig 15-4 Oral manifestations of diabetes.

Q: How should diabetic patients be managed?

- Ask the patients about their blood sugar values.
- Ask them to bring in their hemoglobin A_{1c} lab values.
- If the values are too high, a medical consult should be obtained (regarding changing the type or dosage of medication).
- Be aware that these patients have poor wound healing and must be monitored for a possible medical emergency (see chapter 18).

Q: How can hyperglycemia lead to a diabetic coma?

Figure 15-5 describes the process by which hyperglycemia can lead to a diabetic coma.

Fig 15-5 Process by which hyperglycemia leads to a diabetic coma.

Q: What are the possible macrovascular and microvascular complications of diabetes?

The macrovascular and microvascular complications of diabetes are presented in Fig 15-6.

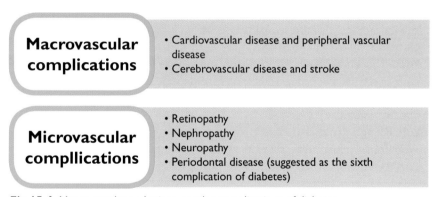

Fig 15-6 Macrovascular and microvascular complications of diabetes.

Organs and Their Functions

Q: Describe the functions of selected body organs.

Pancreas
- Alpha cells produce glucagon (converts glycogen to glucose)
- Beta cells produce insulin and amylin
- Delta cells produce somatostatin (growth hormone)
- Acini produce digestive enzymes (eg, trypsin)

Adrenal gland
- Adrenal cortex secretes corticosteroids (eg, testosterone and aldosterone)
- Adrenal medulla releases catecholamines (eg, tyrosine)

Thyroid
- Involved in metabolism
- Produces calcitonin, which plays a role in calcium homeostasis

Spleen
- White pulp: Active in immune response
- Red pulp: Filters red blood cells

Kidneys
- Creatinine clearance
- Activate vitamin D
- Essential in the urinary system and also serve homeostatic functions such as the regulation of electrolytes, maintenance of acid-base balance, and regulation of blood pressure
- Serve as a natural filter of the blood and remove wastes, which are diverted to the urinary bladder
- Produce hormones including calcitriol and erythropoietin and the enzyme renin

Stomach
- Gastrin, a peptide hormone, stimulates secretion of gastric acid (HCl) by the parietal cells of the stomach and aids in gastric motility.
- Gastric inhibitory peptide decreases both gastric acid release and motility.
- Pepsin, an enzyme whose zymogen (pepsinogen) is released by the chief cells in the stomach, degrades food into peptides.

Anterior pituitary gland
- Luteinizing hormone (LH) is produced by the anterior pituitary gland. In women, an acute rise of LH triggers ovulation and development of the corpus luteum. In men, it stimulates Leydig cell production of testosterone.

• Follicle-stimulating hormone (FSH) is a hormone found in humans and other animals. FSH regulates the development, growth, pubertal maturation, and reproductive processes of the body. FSH and LH act synergistically in reproduction.

Blood

Q: **What is the mechanism of action of warfarin? Heparin?**

• Warfarin: Also known as *coumadin*, warfarin inhibits the vitamin K–dependent synthesis of biologically active forms of the calcium-dependent clotting factors II, VII, IX, and X
• Heparin: Heparin binds to the enzyme inhibitor antithrombin III, causing a conformational change that results in its activation through an increase in the flexibility of its reactive site loop. The activated antithrombin then inactivates thrombin and other proteases involved in blood clotting, most notably factor Xa.

Q: **What patients are most often treated with anticoagulants?**

The patients most often given anticoagulants are those with:

• Atrial fibrillation
• Valvular heart disease
• Mechanical heart valves
• MI
• Recurrent systemic embolism

Q: **What is the difference between prothrombin time (PT) and partial prothrombin time (PTT)?**

Figure 15-7 presents the differences between PT and PTT.

PT	PTT
• Measures the extrinsic pathway of coagulation. • Measures factors I, II, V, VII, and X. • The reference range is usually around 10 to 13 seconds.	• Measures the intrinsic pathway of coagulation. • Typically between 25 and 39 seconds. • Normal PTT times require the presence of the following coagulation factors: I, II, V, VIII, IX, X, XI, and XII. Notably, deficiencies in factors VII or XIII will not be detected with the PTT test.

Fig 15-7 Differences between PT and PTT.

Q: **What is Plavix used for?**

Plavix (Bristol-Myers Squibb/Sanofi) keeps blood platelets from sticking to-gether and forming clots.

Q: **Can patients be removed from antiplatelet therapy for surgery?**

In a science advisory from the American Heart Association and other medical associations, Grines et al[9] stated that a prospective study involving patients taking aspirin or a placebo and undergoing single-tooth extractions showed no statistical difference in postoperative bleeding between the groups. Moreover, they pointed out the lack of well-documented cases of dental procedures, in-cluding multiple tooth extractions, leading to clinical significant postoperative bleeding. The advisory also emphasized that 12 months of dual antiplatelet therapy is essential following the placement of a drug-eluting stent, stating that both patients and health care providers should be made aware of the hazards of premature discontinuation. Finally, it advocates postponing elective surgery for 1 year in high-risk patients with drug-eluting stents or, if that is not possible, continuing aspirin therapy during the perioperative period.

Immune System

Q: **What are the five major classes of immunoglobulin (Ig)?**

1. IgA
2. IgD
3. IgE
4. IgG
5. IgM

See chapter 14 (page 198) for descriptions of the five major classes of Ig.

Q: **Describe the host defense against plaque.**

The host defense against plaque[7] is presented in Fig 15-8.

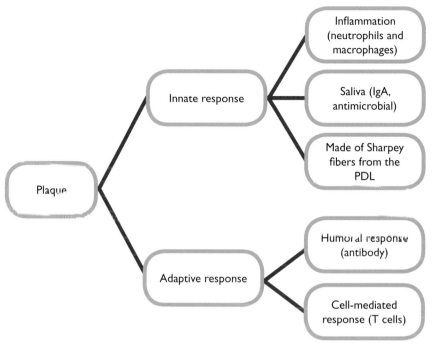

Fig 15-8 Host defense against plaque. PDL—periodontal ligament.

Miscellaneous

Q: **What are the signs and symptoms of liver disease?**

• Jaundice and yellow conjunctiva
• Tender and shrunken liver (accumulation of fluids)
• Peripheral edema
• Prolonged PT

Q: **What are some of the causes and treatment of oral malodor?**

Causes
• Bacteria (most common cause)
• Volatile sulfide compounds
• Gastrointestinal tract problems
• Deep caries, purulent discharge
• Denture left in the mouth overnight

Treatment

- Chlorhexidine 0.12%
- Good oral hygiene regimen
- Referral to medical doctor
- Metal salt solution

Q: What precautions should be taken for a patient who is pregnant?

- According to Huebner et al,[10] comprehensive dental care should be provided during pregnancy not only to prevent pregnancy-specific oral health problems for the mother but also to prevent early childhood caries.
- The best time to treat a pregnant patient is in the second trimester.[11]
- It is a good idea to contact the medical doctor by fax with the treatment plan, including the drugs to be used, quantity, and dosage.
- Tetracycline, vancomycin, and streptomycin should not be used.
- Radiographs should be limited.
- According to the California Dental Association,[12] periodontal treatment is safe for the mother and fetus and has not been shown to cause preterm labor or low birth weight.

References

1. Malamed S. Medical Emergencies in the Dental Office, ed 5. St Louis: Mosby, 2000:34.
2. Burket LW, Greenberg MS, Glick M. Burket's Oral Medicine: Diagnosis and Treatment, ed 10. Hamilton, Ontario: Decker, 2003:14.
3. Humphrey LL, Fu R, Buckley DI, Freeman M, Helfand M. Periodontal disease and coronary heart disease incidence: A systematic review and meta-analysis. J Gen Intern Med 2008;23:2079–2086.
4. Bahekar AA, Singh S, Saha S, Molnar J, Arora R. The prevalence and incidence of coronary heart disease is significantly increased in periodontitis: A meta-analysis. Am Heart J 2007;154:830–837.
5. Beck JD, Offenbacher S, Williams R, Gibbs P, Garcia R. Periodontitis: A risk factor for coronary heart disease? Ann Periodontol 1998;3:127–141.
6. DeStefano F, Anda RF, Kahn HS, Williamson DF, Russell CM. Dental disease and risk of coronary heart disease and mortality. BMJ 1993;306:688–691.
7. Clerehugh V, Tugnait A, Genco RJ. Periodontology at a Glance. Oxford: Wiley-Blackwell, 2009.
8. Friedewald VE, Kornman KS, Beck JD, et al. The American Journal of Cardiology and Journal of Periodontology editors' consensus: Periodontitis and atherosclerotic cardiovascular disease. J Periodontol 2009;80:1021–1032.
9. Grines CL, Bonow RO, Casey DE Jr, et al. Prevention of premature discontinuation of dual antiplatelet therapy in patients with coronary artery stents: A science advisory from the American Heart Association, American College of Cardiology, Society for Cardiovascular Angiography and Interventions, American College of Surgeons, and American Dental Association, with representation from the American College of Physicians. J Am Dent Assoc 2007;138:652–655.
10. Huebner CE, Milgrom P, Conrad D, Lee RS. Providing dental care to pregnant patients: A survey of Oregon general dentists. J Am Dent Assoc 2009;140:211–222.
11. Task Force on Periodontal Treatment of Pregnant Women of the American Academy of Periodontology. American Academy of Periodontology statement regarding periodontal management of the pregnant patient. J Periodontol 2004;75:495.
12. CDA Foundation publishes guidelines for dental care during pregnancy. J Calif Dent Assoc 2010;38:85,87.

Oral Pathology

Staging System for Tumors

Q: Describe the TNM staging system for tumors.

T (size or direct extent of the primary tumor)
- T0: No signs of tumor
- Tis: Carcinoma in situ
- T1: Tumor is less than 2 cm
- T2: Tumor is 2 to 4 cm
- T3: Tumor is greater than 4 cm
- T4: Tumor invades adjacent structures

N (degree of spread to regional lymph nodes)
- N0: Tumor cells absent from regional lymph nodes/not palpable
- N1: Regional lymph node metastasis present (at some sites: tumor spread to closest or small number of regional lymph nodes)
- N2: Tumor spread to an extent between N1 and N3
- N3: Tumor spread to more distant or numerous regional lymph nodes and palpable

M (presence of metastasis)
- M0: No distant metastasis
- M1: Metastasis to distant organs (beyond regional lymph nodes)

Biopsies

Q: What are important rules to know when performing biopsies?

- Biopsy of lesion smaller than 1 cm: Excisional biopsy (removal of the whole lesion)
- Biopsy of lesion greater than 1 cm: Incisional biopsy (surgical removal of part of the lesion; can be done with a biopsy punch)
- Always biopsy a part of the normal tissue around the lesion
- Never perform an incisional biopsy of a pigmented lesion
- Try to put the specimen in a formalin solution

Ulcers and Cysts

Q: What are aphthous ulcers (also known as *canker sores*)?

Aphthous ulcers are painful superficial ulcers of the oral gland-bearing mucosa.[1] They may occur from a deficiency of vitamin B_{12} or folic acid, anemia, or inflammatory bowel syndrome.[2]

Q: What is the treatment for aphthous ulcers?

Chlorhexidine rinses have shown short-term relief in some patients. Vitamin supplements have also been shown to be helpful. Oral lesions may need topical steroid application such as Kenalog (Bristol-Myers Squibb) or Lidex (Medicis Pharmaceutical).

Q: What is the difference between aphthous ulcers and herpetic lesions?

Table 16-1 presents the differences between aphthous ulcers and herpetic lesions. A cytologic smear can be performed to rule out a viral etiology.[3]

Table 16-1 | Aphthous ulcers and herpetic lesions

	Aphthous ulcers	Herpetic lesions
Movement	Movable	Bound
Area found	Mucosa	Keratinized and gland-bearing tissue
Coalescence	Do not coalesce	Coalesce
Forms	Major (> 1 cm) / minor (< 1 cm) / herpetiform (may be on keratinized mucosa)	Primary/recurrent

Q: What is the treatment for herpetic lesions?

5% acyclovir cream can shorten the duration of the episode. 1% penciclovir was shown to be more effective than 5% acyclovir in reducing the healing time and duration of the painful phase.[4]

The lesions are self-limiting and run a course of 7 to 14 days.[3]

Q: Describe the lateral periodontal cyst and the odontogenic keratocyst.

Characteristics of the lateral periodontal cyst and the odontogenic keratocyst are presented in Fig 16-1.

Lateral periodontal cyst	Odontogenic keratocyst
• An odontogenic cyst derived from rests of the dental lamina. • It is most often found in the mandibular premolar region. • The treatment is enucleation.	• Also derived from rests of dental lamina. • It is a cyst that occurs most often in the posterior body and ramus area. • It is one of the features of nevoid basal cell carcinoma. • It is treated by surgical enucleation.

Fig 16-1 Characteristics of the lateral periodontal cyst and the odontogenic keratocyst.

Epithelial Disorders

Q: Describe pseudoepitheliomatous hyperplasia.

Pseudoepitheliomatous hyperplasia is increased cell production of the squamous epithelium that is similar to squamous cell carcinoma. It is seen in chronic candidiasis and papillary hyperplasia.

Q: What is leukoplakia?

Leukoplakia is a clinical term used to denote mucosal conditions that produce coloration of the mucous membranes that is whiter than normal. It has been found to turn to squamous cell carcinoma 5.4% of the time. It is usually found in the buccal mucosa.[1]

Q: What is proliferative verrucous leukoplakia?

Proliferative verrucous leukoplakia is an uncommon leukoplakia that creates papillary areas of epithelial hyperplasia that have the potential to develop into verrucous or squamous cell carcinoma. The treatment of choice is local incision.

Q: **What is erythroplakia?**

Erythroplakia is a painless, red, velvety, and plaque-like lesion of the mucous membranes that does not rub off. It is caused by epithelial dysplasia, carcinoma in situ, or squamous cell carcinoma. Histologic analysis shows that 60% to 90% of erythroplakias are epithelial dysplasia, carcinoma in situ, or squamous cell carcinoma.[1] It usually occurs on the floor of the mouth, ventral tongue, and soft palate. Depending on the stage, these lesions are usually excised.

Q: **What is the most common malignant neoplasm of the oral cavity? What are its causes?**

Squamous cell carcinoma represents 90% of all oral cancers. It is most often seen on the lower lip, lateral and ventral areas of the tongue, and the floor of the mouth. The causes are illustrated in Fig 16-2.

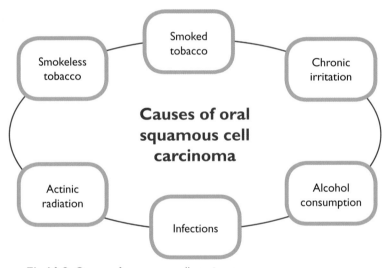

Fig 16-2 Causes of squamous cell carcinoma.

Q: **How is squamous cell carcinoma treated?**

Depending on the stage, it is usually treated by excision, radiation, or both.

Q: **What sites metastasize to the mouth?**

The kidney, skin, and lungs metastasize to the mouth.

Q: **Explain the ABCDE staging system for skin cancer.**

The ABCDE staging system for skin cancer is presented in Fig 16-3.

A	Asymmetric
B	Border: Not well defined
C	Color: Not uniform
D	Diameter: Larger than a pencil eraser (6 mm)
E	Elevation: Raised or irregular surface

Fig 16-3 ABCDE staging for skin cancer.

Connective Tissue Lesions

Q: Describe a pyogenic granuloma.

A *pyogenic granuloma* is a small, fast-growing rounded mass of inflamed tissue made of endothelial cells usually found on the gingiva. They are also known as pregnancy tumors because they often occur during the second and third trimesters of pregnancy. The lesion should be excised and curetted.

Q: What is a giant cell fibroma?

A *giant cell fibroma* is a reactive fibrous proliferation. It is called a *giant cell fibroma* because of binucleated and trinucleated fibroblasts that occur in close proximity to the epithelium. Local excision is the treatment of choice.

Q: Describe inflammatory papillary hyperplasia.

Inflammatory papillary hyperplasia is an overgrowth of fibrous connective tissue beneath a loose or ill-fitting denture. Usually the chronic inflammation is confined to the palatal vault. The hyperplastic tissue needs to be removed before a new denture is made.

Odontogenic Tumors

Q: What is the difference between a compound and a complex odontoma?

An odontoma is found predominantly in young adults and contains enamel, dentin, pulp, and cementum. A *compound odontoma* is tooth shaped and found in the anterior of the mouth. A *complex odontoma* is a solid mass and found in the posterior of the mouth. Treatment is enucleation.

Q: Describe the characteristics of an ameloblastoma.

An *ameloblastoma* is a slow-growing and aggressive tumor with a broad spectrum of histologic features. It is multicystic, has a soap bubble appearance on radiographs, and occurs most frequently in the mandible. It is rare for an ameloblastoma to metastasize. Treatment is marginal or block resection due to their high recurrence rate.

Immune-Mediated Disorders

Q: What is desquamative gingivitis?

Desquamative gingivitis is characterized by scooped-out gingiva, diffuse gingival erythema, and mucosal sloughing and erosion. It is found in lichen planus, pemphigus vulgaris, mucous membrane pemphigoid, and lupus.

Q: Describe the differences between pemphigus vulgaris and mucous membrane pemphigoid.

The differences between pemphigus vulgaris and mucous membrane pemphigoid are shown in Fig 16-4.

Pemphigus vulgaris	• Autoimmune reaction to desmosomes above the basal layer • Fishnet appearance revealed in immunofluorescence • Tzanck cells • Higher incidence in Ashkenazi Jewish population • Treatment: Prednisolone (150 to 360 mg) daily for 6 to 8 weeks
Mucous membrane pemphigoid	• Autoimmune reaction occurs at the level of the basement membrane affecting the hemidesmosomes • Smooth line appearance revealed in immunofluorescence • Associated with cicatricial pemphigoid and bullous pemphigoid • Treatment: Combination of systemic and topical steroids

Fig 16-4 Characteristics of pemphigus vulgaris and mucous membrane pemphigoid.

Q: What is the Nikolsky test?

The *Nikolsky test* consists of rubbing the tissue with a blunt instrument and observing whether a blister forms in minutes. Blister formation indicates that the clinical test is positive. The test is positive in patients with disorders in cell cohesion at the basement membrane (eg, mucous membrane pemphigoid).

Q: What is erythema multiforme?

Erythema multiforme is a hypersensitivity reaction that is centered on superficial vessels of the skin and is of immune origin. It clinically presents as ulcerations on any mucosal site, and it is most common in young adult men. The immunofluorescent pattern is perivascular. It can be incited by the following:

- Drugs (penicillin and sulfa)
- Gastrointestinal conditions (Crohn disease and ulcerative colitis)
- Infections (herpes)
- Vaccinations

Treatment is to find the inciting factor and neutralize it. The condition is usually self-limiting.

Q: Describe lichen planus.

Lichen planus is an inflammatory disease that can appear as a white reticular plaque or as an erosive lesion with a noticeable T lymphocyte reaction in the connective tissue. The chance for malignant transformation is 0.4% to 2%. The immunofluorescent pattern is shaggy on the basement membrane. There are three forms, which are described in Table 16-2.

Table 16-2 | Forms of lichen planus

	Reticular	Erosive	Plaque
Description	Wickham striae: raised, thin, white lines that have a reticular pattern	Painful erythematous or white pseudomembranous areas	White raised or flattened area
Most common area of the mouth	Buccal mucosa, tongue, and gingiva	Buccal mucosa, tongue, and gingiva	Tongue

Q: Describe the characteristics of lupus erythematosus.

Lupus erythematosus is an autoimmune disorder with chronic inflammation of the skin, connective tissues, and internal organs. It is commonly found in middle-aged women. It is thought that antibodies target DNA. It is characterized in the mouth with buccomucosal lesions. It is usually treated with topical steroids, antimalarial agents, and sulfones.

Q: What are some preventive treatments to consider for patients with Sjögren syndrome?

Sjögren syndrome is a chronic autoimmune disease that attacks the exocrine glands that produce tears and saliva. Maintenance is as follows:

- Four-month recall: 1.23% acidulated phosphate sodium fluoride gel in a fluoride tray for 4 minutes or 2.25% fluoride varnish
- Patient should brush with a fluoride dentifrice (Prevident 5000 Plus, Colgate-Palmolive)
- Chlorhexidine 0.12% rinse for 30 seconds at night

Salivary Gland Disorders

Q: What is the difference between a mucocele and a mucus retention cyst?

Table 16-3 presents the defining characteristics of mucoceles and mucus retention cysts.

Table 16-3 Characteristics of mucoceles and mucus retention cysts

	Mucocele	Mucus retention cyst
Definition	Swelling in the mouth when a salivary duct is severed	Cyst caused by an obstruction of a duct
Lining	Granulation tissue	Lined by epithelium
Common location	Lower lip	Lower lip and buccal mucosa
Differential	Mucus retention cyst, fibroma, neuroma, and mucoepidermoid carcinoma	Mucocele and mucoepidermoid carcinoma

Oral Infections

Q: How does herpes zoster manifest itself in the oral cavity?

Herpes zoster can appear as a vesicular eruption on the mucosa as well as on the skin. The lesions can arise along the ophthalmic, maxillary, and mandibular distribution of the nerve. Herpes zoster can be very painful.

Q: Describe the features of necrotizing ulcerative periodontitis (an extension of necrotizing ulcerative gingivitis).

Necrotizing ulcerative periodontitis is a necrotizing disease that extends to the gingiva and bone. The features of necrotizing ulcerative periodontitis[5] are presented in Fig 16-5.

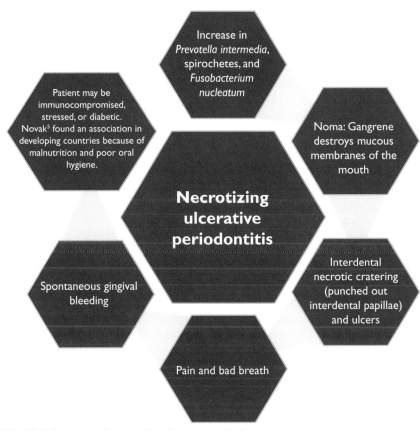

Fig 16-5 Features of necrotizing ulcerative periodontitis.

Q: What is the treatment for necrotizing ulcerative periodontitis?

Treatment consists of chlorhexidine, metronidazole (250 mg taken four times per day), and local debridement. Novak[5] noted that adjunctive systemic metronidazole therapy has been shown to effectively manage human immunodeficiency virus (HIV)–associated periodontitis and control spirochetal infection but warned of the risk of superinfection with oral *Candida* associated with the use of systemic antibiotics, particularly in the treatment of patients with HIV.

Q: Describe the symptoms of atrophic candidiasis.

• Most commonly found on the palate under a denture
• A continuous painful burning feeling
• Increased sensitivity

Papillon-Lèfevre Syndrome

Q: **Describe Papillon-Lèfevre syndrome.**

Papillon-Lèfevre syndrome is an autosomal recessive disorder caused by deficiency of cathepsin C. Severe periodontal disease affects the primary teeth (by 4 years of age, most of the primary teeth are lost) and permanent teeth (by 14 years of age, most of the permanent teeth are lost).[1] There is also hyperkeratosis of the palms of the hands and soles of the feet.

Differential Diagnosis

Q: **What is the differential diagnosis for a bump?**

The differential diagnosis for a bump includes:

- Fibroma
- Traumatic neuroma
- Neurofibroma
- Giant cell fibroma
- Peripheral fibroma
- Peripheral ossifying fibroma
- Giant cell fibroma
- Traumatic neuroma
- Pyogenic granuloma
- Periodontal abscess (parulis)
- Ranula
- Lymphangioma
- Salivary gland enlargement
- Lipoma
- Leiomyoma
- Rhabdomyoma
- Hemangioma
- Granular cell tumor
- Schwannoma

Q: **What is the differential diagnosis for a circumscribed flat lesion? Circumscribed elevated lesion?**

Flat
- Ephelis
- Junctional nevus
- Café au lait spots or macules
- Lentigo
- Melanotic macule

Elevated
- Nevi
- Seborrheic keratosis
- Melanoma

Q: What is the differential diagnosis for a nonspecific ulcer?

- Aphthae
- Squamous cell carcinoma
- Herpetic ulcer
- Traumatic ulcer
- Traumatic granuloma
- Primary/secondary syphilis
- Necrotizing ulcerative gingivitis
- Herpangina

Q: What is the differential diagnosis for a pericoronal radiolucency?

- Dentigerous cyst
- Odontogenic keratocyst
- Ameloblastoma

Q: What are the differential diagnoses for pigmented, white, and red lesions?

Figure 16-6 presents the differential diagnoses for pigmented, white, and red lesions.

Pigmented lesions	White lesions	Red lesions
• Amalgam tattoo	• Epithelial hyperplasia	• Squamous cell carcinoma
• Mucosal nevi	• Frictional keratosis	• Erythematous *Candida*
• Vascular malformation	• Plaque-type lichen planus	• Contact stomatitis
• Melanotic macule	• Chronic hyperplastic *Candida*	• Drug reaction
• Melanoma	• Tobacco-related leukoplakia	• Geographic tongue (Fig 16-8)
• Blue nevus	• Hairy leukoplakia	• Osteosarcoma
• Kaposi sarcoma	• Snuff dipper's pouch (Fig 16-7)	• Ecchymosis
• Black hairy tongue	• Hyperkeratosis	• Kaposi sarcoma
	• Squamous cell carcinoma	• Angular cheilitis
	• Proliferative verrucous leukoplakia	• Erythroplakia
	• Leukoedema	• Atrophic glossitis
	• Fordyce granules	

Fig 16-6 Differential diagnoses for pigmented, white, and red lesions.

Fig 16-7 Snuff dipper's pouch in the anterior area of the mouth from chewing smokeless tobacco.

Fig 16-8 Geographic tongue.

Q: What is the differential diagnosis for a papillary lesion?

The differential diagnosis for a papillary lesion[3] includes:

- Oral papilloma
- Verruca vulgaris
- Verrucas carcinoma
- Squamous papilloma
- Inflammatory papillary hyperplasia
- Condyloma acuminatum
- Focal epithelial hyperplasia

Q: What is the differential diagnosis for a lump in the midline of the neck? Lateral neck?

The differential diagnoses for a lump in the midline of the neck and in the lateral neck are presented in Fig 16-9.

Midline of the neck
- Thyroglossal duct cyst
- Thyroiditis
- Goiter
- Thyroid tumors
- Hashimoto disease

Lateral neck
- Branchial cleft cyst
- Lymphadenitis
- Hodgkin and Non-Hodgkin lymphoma

Fig 16-9 Differential diagnoses for a lump in the midline and lateral region of the neck.

Miscellaneous

Q: What is the difference between osteogenesis imperfecta and dentinogenesis imperfecta?

Table 16-4 presents the characteristics of osteogenesis imperfecta and dentogenesis imperfecta.

Table 16-4	Osteogenesis imperfecta (OI) and dentinogenesis imperfecta (DI)	
	Osteogenesis imperfecta	**Dentinogenesis imperfecta**
Definition	• Alteration in formation of bone • Inability of the matrix to mineralize	Undermineralized dentin obliterates pulp chambers and canals
Characteristics	Blue sclera	• Opalescent teeth • Dentin is soft
Treatment	Orthopedic treatment is usually nonsurgical	Appropriate restorations are made to prevent further loss of enamel
Relation to one another	25% have DI	Type 1: Patients have OI Type 2: Patients do not have OI Type 3: Mostly in Maryland, primary teeth have multiple pulp exposures

Q: What is the difference between actinic cheilitis and angular cheilitis?

Table 16-5 presents the characteristics and treatment of actinic cheilitis and angular cheilitis.

Table 16-5	Definition and treatment of actinic cheilitis and angular cheilitis	
	Actinic cheilitis	**Angular cheilitis**
Definition	• Red and white patches with telangiectasia • Caused by prolonged exposure to sunlight • Premalignant squamous cell carcinoma occurs in 10% of cases	• Bilateral fissures at the corners of the mouth usually caused by *Candida albicans* • May have secondary infection with bacteria
Treatment	Superficial surgical removal of the damaged tissue unless metastasis has occurred	Antifungal ointment alone or in combination with antibiotics

Q: What is PFAPA syndrome?

Periodic fever, aphthous stomatitis, pharyngitis, and adenitis or *periodic fever aphthous pharyngitis and cervical adenopathy* (PFAPA) syndrome is a medical condition, typically starting in young children, in which high fever occurs periodically at intervals of about 3 to 5 weeks, frequently accompanied by aphthous ulcers, pharyngitis, or adenitis. A possible treatment is a dose of prednisone.

Q: What are the comorbidities found in patients with AIDS?

- Hairy leukoplakia
- *Candida*/angular cheilitis
- Atrophic *Candida*
- Kaposi sarcoma
- Non-Hodgkin lymphoma
- Linear gingivitis
- Herpes simplex/herpes zoster

Q: What is mucoepidermoid carcinoma?

Mucoepidermoid carcinoma is the most common salivary gland carcinoma and the malignant tumor most frequently found in individuals younger than 20 years. It does not have a capsule and is composed of mucus-secreting and stratified squamous epithelial cells. About two-thirds of mucoepidermoid carcinomas are found within the parotid gland; the remaining one-third are located within the minor salivary glands.[6] The treatment is based on its grade. If it is found in the parotid gland, lobectomy and cervical node dissection are indicated if the nodes are palpable.

Q: Do cemento-osseous lesions need to be treated?

Cemento-osseous lesions, which are common in the black population, do not need to be treated. They consist of calcifications at the apices of the teeth, and patients have no symptoms.

References

1. Sapp JP, Eversole LR, Wysocki GP. Contemporary Oral and Maxillofacial Pathology, ed 2. St Louis: Mosby, 2004:40,174,183,253.
2. Woo SB, Sonis ST. Recurrent aphthous ulcers: A review of diagnosis and treatment. J Am Dent Assoc 1996;127:1202–1213.
3. Newland JR, Meiller TF, Wynn RL, Crossley HL. Oral Soft Tissue Diseases: A Reference Manual for Diagnosis and Management, ed 2. Hudson, Ohio: Lexi-Comp, 2002:29,48,53,87.
4. Snoeck R. Antiviral therapy of herpes simplex. Int J Antimicrob Agents 2000;16:157–159.
5. Novak MJ. Necrotizing ulcerative periodontitis. Ann Periodontol 1999;4:74–78.
6. Mucoepidermoid Carcinoma. http://www.thedoctorsdoctor.com/diseases/mucoepidermoid_ca.htm. Accessed 2 October 2012.

Lasers

Background

Q: What is *laser* an acronym for?

Laser stands for *l*ight *a*mplification by *s*timulated *e*mission of *r*adiation.

Q: What are the most common types of lasers used in periodontics?

The most common types of laser used in periodontics[1] are presented in Fig 17-1.

Carbon dioxide (CO$_2$)	Neodyminium: yttrium-aluminum-garnet (Nd:YAG)	Erbium:yttrium-aluminum-garnet (Er:YAG)
• 10,600-nm wavelength • Useful for soft tissue surgery such as frenectomy, degranulation, biopsy, and gingivectomy	• 1,064-nm wavelength • Affinity for pigmented colors and can penetrate deep beyond the surface • Useful for soft tissue incision, subgingival ablation, and bacterial elimination	• 2,940-nm wavelength for the free-running laser • Useful for soft tissue incision and ablation, subgingival curettage, scaling of root surfaces, osteoplasty and ostectomy • Highly absorbed in both water and hydroxyapatite

Fig 17-1 Types of lasers.

Q: What are the advantages and disadvantages of lasers?

Figure 17-2 presents the advantages and disadvantages of lasers.[2–4]

Advantages	Disadvantages
• Relatively bloodless • Minimal swelling and scarring • Coagulation • Minimal suturing • Less postsurgical pain	• Minimal evidence for use as a monotherapy • Not been shown to be better than scaling and root planing • May have delayed scar contraction (wound healing) • Expensive • There is potential for root surface damage (especiallly Er:YAG) • May reach the patient's eyes (need to prevent irradiation to eyes)

Fig 17-2 Advantages and disadvantages of lasers.

Different Types of Laser Therapies

Q: What is photodynamic therapy?

Photodynamic therapy unites low-level laser light with a photosensitizer (a nontoxic dye), which attaches to the target cells and destroys microorganisms.[1]

Q: What is the laser-assisted new attachment procedure (LANAP)?

LANAP (Millennium Dental Technologies) uses the Nd:YAG laser to remove the pocket epithelium and necrotic epithelium; however, the connective tissue is spared, allowing healing and regeneration to occur. The manufacturer claims decreased postoperative bleeding and recession compared with conventional osseous surgery.

Effectiveness

Q: Have lasers been found to be effective in treating chronic periodontitis?

Cobb's review[4] found that in terms of reducing pocket depth and subgingival bacterial populations, Nd:YAG and Er:YAG lasers have been shown to be as effective as scaling and root planing (SRP) in the treatment of chronic peri-

odontitis. However, he described the evidence for laser therapy being superior to traditional nonsurgical periodontal therapy in regard to gain in clinical
attachment level (the "gold standard") as "minimal at best." Karlsson et al[5] did
not find consistent evidence to support the effectiveness of adjunctive laser
treatment in adults with chronic periodontitis.

Q: Are lasers more effective than traditional SRP?

A statement by the American Academy of Periodontology[3] reported "minimal
evidence" supporting the use of lasers as a monotherapy or adjunctively with
SRP for subgingival debridement. It went on to state that although in vitro
studies have shown the Er:YAG laser to remove calculus and to negate endotoxin, there is a risk of damage to the root surface during calculus removal
due to the inability of the laser operator to see the area being lased by the
hard tissue laser. It concluded that on the whole lasers have been shown to
be "unpredictable and inconsistent in their ability to reduce subgingival microbial loads" to a greater degree than SRP alone.

Cobb[4] found limited proof that lasers used in an adjunctive capacity to SRP
may offer some further benefit.

Eberhard et al[6] found that, although the efficacy of Er:YAG did not reach
that achieved by hand instrumentation, it was capable of removing calculus
from periodontally involved root surfaces. He also found that, opposed to
scaling and root planing, the lack of cementum removal may qualify the laser
as a different approach during supportive periodontal therapy.

In Slot et al's review[7] of initial treatment of periodontitis, they found that
studies confirmed no beneficial effect for a pulsed Nd:YAG laser compared
with conventional therapy.

Q: Can lasers be used for crown lengthening?

Presently, there are no controlled longitudinal or cohort studies demonstrating the use of lasers for clinical crown lengthening using the closed-flap technique.[4]

Q: Is photodynamic therapy effective?

Braham et al[8] found that antimicrobial photodynamic therapy may enhance the outcomes of periodontal treatment through its bactericidal activity and ability to inactivate bacterial virulence factors and host cytokines that impede healing. Berakdar et al[1] demonstrated a slightly higher improvement of clinical parameters with photodynamic therapy in addition to SRP than with SRP alone.

Azarpazhooh et al[9] demonstrated in a meta-analysis that photodynamic therapy as an independent treatment or as an adjunct to SRP was not superior to SRP alone and as a result did not recommend photodynamic therapy to routinely treat periodontitis. According to a statement by the American Academy of Periodontology,[3] photodynamic therapy is arbitrary and variable.

Q: Is LANAP successful?

In a statement regarding the use of dental lasers for excisional new attachment procedures (ENAP), the American Academy of Periodontology[10] states that there is a lack of evidence that "laser ENAP" or "laser curettage" provides clinical advantages in terms of treatment results compared with traditional periodontal therapy. They also point to evidence suggesting that such use of lasers could interfere with normal cell attachment and healing on root surfaces and adjacent alveolar bone.

Yukna et al[11] found that LANAP-treated teeth displayed superior probing depth reductions and clinical probing attachment level gains compared with control teeth. New cementum and new connective tissue attachment was observed on all teeth treated with LANAP.

Safety

Q: Can lasers be used around dental implants?

Wilcox et al[12] studied the Nd:YAG laser and found that prudent use of the laser unit yields temperature profiles within clinical parameters in the presence of dental implants.

Galli et al[13] recommended operating Er:YAG lasers with care on titanium surfaces based on evidence that the laser may reduce the viability and the activity of osteoblastic cells.

Romanos et al[14] studied the CO_2 laser and observed osteoblast growth on titanium surfaces. The study concluded that osteoblast attachment and bone formation may be fostered by laser irradiation of titanium surfaces.

Q: Is there potential for root surface damage with the Er:YAG laser?

According to a statement by the American Academy of Periodontology,[3] there is a risk of damage to the root surface during calculus removal by Er:YAG laser due to the inability of the operator to see the area being lased by the hard tissue laser.

References

1. Berakdar M, Callaway A, Eddin MF, Ross A, Willershausen B. Comparison between scaling-root-planing (SRP) and SRP/photodynamic therapy: Six-month study. Head Face Med 2012;8:12.
2. Pick RM, Colvard MD. Current status of lasers in soft tissue dental surgery. J Periodontol 1993;64:589–602.
3. American Academy of Periodontology statement on the efficacy of lasers in the non-surgical treatment of inflammatory periodontal disease. J Periodontol 2011;82:513–514.
4. Cobb CM. Lasers in periodontics: A review of the literature. J Periodontol 2006;77:545–564.
5. Karlsson MR, Diogo Löfgren CI, Jansson HM. The effect of laser therapy to nonsurgical periodontal treatment in subjects with chronic periodontitis: A systematic review. J Periodontol 2008;79:2021–2028.
6. Eberhard J, Ehlers H, Falk W, Açil Y, Albers HK, Jepsen S. Efficacy of subgingival calculus removal with Er:YAG laser compared to mechanical debridement: An in situ study. J Clin Periodontol 2003;30:511–518.
7. Slot DE, Kranendonk AA, Paraskevas S, Van der Weijden F. The effect of a pulsed Nd:YAG laser in nonsurgical periodontal therapy. J Periodontol 2009;80:1041–1056.
8. Braham P, Herron C, Street C, Darveau R. Antimicrobial photodynamic therapy may promote periodontal healing through multiple mechanisms. J Periodontol 2009;80:1790–1798.
9. Azarpazhooh A, Shah PS, Tenenbaum HC, Goldberg MB. The effect of photodynamic therapy for periodontitis: A systematic review and meta-analysis. J Periodontol 2010;81:4–14.
10. American Academy of Periodontology. Statement Regarding Use of Dental Lasers for Excisional New Attachment Procedure (ENAP). http://www.perio.org/resources-products/enap_laser.htm. Accessed 2 October 2012.
11. Yukna RA, Carr RL, Evans GH. Histologic evaluation of an Nd:YAG laser-assisted new attachment procedure in humans. Int J Periodontics Restorative Dent 2007;27:577–587.
12. Wilcox CW, Wilwerding TM, Watson P, Morris JT. Use of electrosurgery and lasers in the presence of dental implants. Int J Oral Maxillofac Implants 2001;16:578–582.
13. Galli C, Macaluso GM, Elezi E, et al. The effects of Er:YAG laser treatment on titanium surface profile and osteoblastic cell activity: An in vitro study. J Periodontol 2011;82:1169–1177.
14. Romanos G, Crespi R, Barone A, Covani U. Osteoblast attachment on titanium disks after laser irradiation. Int J Oral Maxillofac Implants 2006;21:232–236.

Medical Emergencies

Cardiopulmonary Resuscitation (CPR)

Q: Explain how CPR should be performed for patients of all ages.

Table 18-1 presents instructions for performing CPR on patients of different age groups.

Table 18-1	CPR procedure for patients of different age groups*			
	Compression to ventilation ratio		**Compressions**	**Rescue breaths**
	One rescuer	**Two rescuers**		
Adult CPR	30:2	30:2	At least 100 per minute and 2 inches deep	Every 5 seconds for 1 second
Child CPR (ages 1 to 13)	30:2	15:2	At least 100 per minute and 2 inches deep	Every 3 to 5 seconds for 1 second
Infant CPR (0 to 11 months)	30:2	15:2	At least 100 per minute and 1.5 inches deep	Every 3 to 5 seconds for 1 second

*Data from American Academy of CPR and First Aid.[1]

Q: What are the ABCDs of checking an unconscious person?

- Airway
- Breathing
- Circulation
- Definitive treatment

Emergency Drugs

Q: What are some essential drugs to have in the emergency kit?

Figure 18-1 presents drugs that are essential to an emergency kit.

Oxygen: Mobile E tanks	Epinephrine: Already drawn up/epinephrine pen (0.3 to 0.5 mg)	Nitroglycerine (pill or spray): chest pain
Albuterol inhaler: β2 agonist, stops bronchospasm, asthma, and allergy	Benadryl (McNeil): Minor allergy, 50 mg three times per day	Sugar: Hypoglycemia
	Aspirin: Heart attack patients	Spirits of ammonia: Syncope

Fig 18-1 Emergency kit drugs.

Q: What are the secondary drugs that can be helpful in an emergency?

- Nitrous oxide: Pain control for heart attacks
- Glucagon: 1 mg for hypoglycemic patients
- Valium (Roche): Benzodiazepine for epilepsy
- Hydrocortisone: Allergy
- Reversal drugs: Intravenous (IV) sedation

Office Emergencies

Q: **How can the diagnosis of an emergency condition be established?**

Figure 18-2 presents the process of diagnosing a medical emergency.

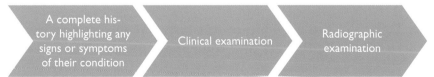

Fig 18-2 Diagnosis of a medical emergency.

Q: **What are the common reasons a patient may lose consciousness and the associated treatments?**

Figure 18-3 presents common reasons a patient may lose consciousness and the treatments associated with each.

Fig 18-3 Causes and treatment of loss of consciousness. IM—intramuscularly.

Q: Describe a grand mal seizure.

Grand mal epilepsy is the most common form of seizure disorder. Causes include drug withdrawal, photic stimulation, menstruation, fatigue, alcohol, falling asleep, or awakening. The seizure could last 5 to 15 minutes.[2]

    Management of the patient includes protecting the airway (remove any objects from their mouth) and preventing the patient from injury. After being monitored, the patient can be discharged to an adult companion or friend.

Q: Describe the possible conditions that may result from respiratory distress and their management.

Management of the conditions that may result from respiratory distress is presented in Fig 18-4.

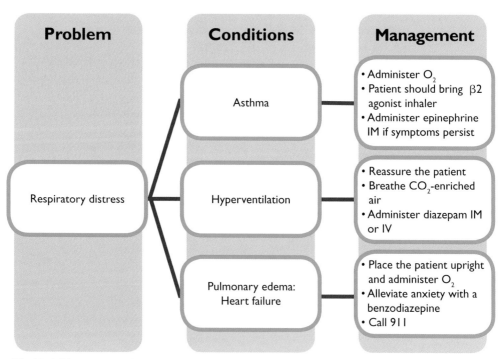

Fig 18-4 Management of conditions resulting from respiratory distress. IM—intramuscularly.

Q: What are some reasons a patient may walk into the office confused?

Figure 18-5 presents possible causes for patient confusion.

Diabetes: May be hypogly-cemic or hyperglycemic	Alcohol or drug overdose
Hyperthyroidism or hypothyroidism	Cerebrovascular incident: Call 911

Fig 18-5 Causes of patient confusion.

Q: What are some reactions a patient may have to local anesthetic administration?

Possible patient reactions to local anesthetic administration include[2]:

- Overdose: Watch patient and check vitals.
- Allergy: Mild—50 mg Benadryl or a histamine blocker intramuscularly (IM); severe—epinephrine (0.3 to 0.5 mg) IM or IV and call 911.
- Hyperventilation: Reassure the patient and allow them to breathe CO_2-enriched air. It may be necessary to administer diazepam IM or IV.

Q: What are some reasons a patient walking into the practice may experience chest pain?

Figure 18-6 presents reasons for chest pain. For angina, a nitroglycerin tablet (0.3 to 0.5 mg) may be given. However, in potential cases of myocardial infarction, a call to 911 needs to be made as aspirin, nitrous oxide, and oxygen are administered.

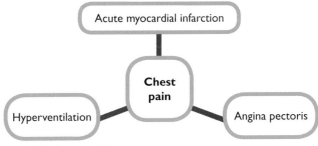

Fig 18-6 Causes of chest pain.

Q: What is the difference between angina and myocardial infarction?

The difference between angina and myocardial infarction is presented in Fig 18-7.

Angina:	Myocardial infarction:
Reversible ischemic damage to myocardium cased by insufficient oxygen to the myocardium and emboli	Irreversible ischemic damage to the myocardium

Fig 18-7 Difference between angina and myocardial infarction.

References

1. American Academy of CPR and First Aid. BLS CPR (Adult / Child / Infant): Summary. http://www. onlinecprcertification.net/free_course.php?id=2&page=2&cid=89&type=ch. Accessed 3 October 2012.

Treatment Planning

Read the case presentations, then answer the questions that follow. Teeth are numbered according to the two-digit FDI notation.

Case 1

Patient identification

- Age: 36 years
- Ethnicity: White

History of present illness

Chief complaint: "My dentist told me to come see a periodontist. I was told that I need gum surgery."

Medical history

- Significant past illnesses: None
- Allergies: None
- Medications: None

Current medical history
- General health: Good
- Head/eyes/ears/nose/throat: None
- Neuromuscular: None
- Respiratory: None
- Cardiovascular: None
- Gastrointestinal: None
- Genitourinary: None
- Hematologic/immune: None

Family history
- Diabetes: None
- Cardiovascular disease: None
- Bleeding disorders: None
- Tuberculosis: None
- Mental/emotional disorders: None
- Periodontal disease: None

Social history
- Diet: Healthy
- Smoking: Past marijuana smoker (12 years)
- Exercise: Seldom
- Alcohol: 1 to 2 drinks/week

Dental history

- Restorative experience: Minimal
- Orthodontics: None reported
- Frequency of prior care: Infrequent
- Oral hygiene: Fair
  - Brushing: Once a day
  - Flossing: Twice a day

Clinical examination

Dental examination
- Missing: 18 and 28 (Fig 19-1a)
- Restorations:
  - 26 distal/occlusal/buccal/lingual: silver
  - 36 distal/occlusal and buccal pit: silver (Fig 19-1b)
  - 46 buccal: silver
- Open contacts: None (Fig 19-1c)
- Wear facets/attrition: Generalized moderate occlusal and incisal wear
- Abrasion: None
- Abfraction: None
- Parafunctional activity: Suspected clenching/grinding
- Marginal ridge discrepancies: 37 and 38; 47 and 48
- Staining: Moderate generalized staining (Figs 19-1d and 19-1e)

Occlusal examination
- Angle classification: Dental molar Class I
- Canine relationship: Class I on the left; edge to edge on the right
- Centric relation: Repeatable
- Left lateral guidance: Lateral anterior guidance
- Right lateral guidance: Lateral anterior guidance
- Protrusive guidance: 11, 21, 31, 32, 41, and 42
- Incisal relationship:
  - Horizontal overlap: 2 mm
  - Vertical overlap: 2 mm
- Fremitus: 12
- Crossbite: None

Fig 19-1 (a) Maxillary occlusal view. (b) Mandibular occlusal view. (c) Frontal view. (d) Lingual view of the maxillary anterior teeth. (e) Facial view of the mandibular anterior teeth.

Periodontal examination (Fig 19-2)

- Plaque/calculus: Generalized plaque accumulation with moderate to heavy supragingival and subgingival calculus
- Oral hygiene: Poor
- Plaque free: 34% (initial)
- Marginal bleeding: 14% (initial)
- Periodontal tissues:
  - Color: Pink with localized areas of erythematous tissue and blunted papillae
  - Texture: Generalized smooth appearance
  - Tone: Generally fibrous and edematous at the gingival margin; interdental papillae are spongy
- Probing depths: Generalized 2 to 7 mm
- Bleeding on probing (BOP): Localized
- Suppuration: 14

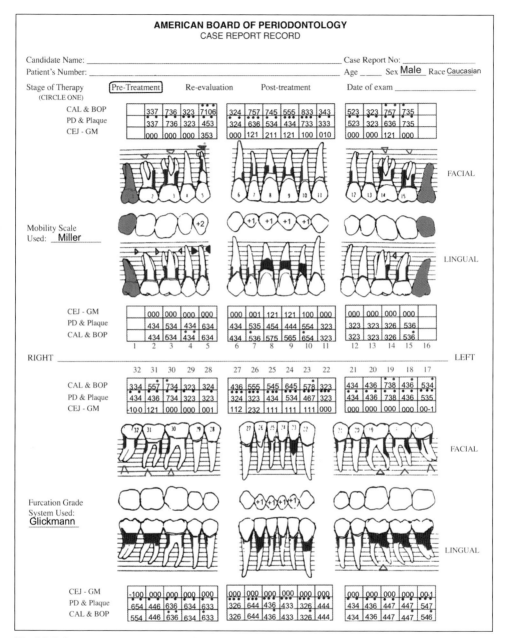

AMERICAN BOARD OF PERIODONTOLOGY
CASE REPORT RECORD

Candidate Name: _____ Case Report No: _____

Patient's Number: _____ Age _____ Sex **Male** Race Caucasian

Stage of Therapy [Pre-Treatment] Re-evaluation Post-treatment Date of exam _____
(CIRCLE ONE)

Mobility Scale Used: **Miller**

Furcation Grade System Used: **Glickmann**

Fig 19-2 Pretreatment report record.

- Recession (Miller):
  - Class 1: 11, 12, 21 to 23, 26, 31, 32, 41 to 44, 47
  - Class 2: 14B
- Mucogingival problems: 14, no keratinized attached tissue
- Vestibular depth: Good vestibular depth except for 38 and 48

Fig 19-3 Pretreatment radiographs.

- Mobility (Miller):
  - Class I: 11, 12, 21, 22, 31, 32, 41, 42
  - Class II: 14
- Furcation (Glickman):
  - Grade I: 27B, 38B, 37B, 47B, and 48B
  - Grade II: 17B, 17DL, 16B, 16ML, 16DL, 26B, 26DL, 36BL, and 46B
  - Grade III: 14BMD
- Anatomical considerations: Thin periodontal biotype, short root trunk, and the sinus is proximal to the maxillary molar roots

Radiographic examination (Fig 19-3)

- Bone loss: Generalized moderate to advanced horizontal bone loss, with localized vertical defects
- Radiographic bone loss:
  - Mesial bone loss: 16, 47
  - Distal bone loss: 17, 48
  - Mesial and distal bone loss: 11, 12, 14, 21, 22, 26, 27, 31, 35 to 38, 41, 42, 46
- Periapical radiolucencies: 14
- Root form: Long and tapering
- Furcation radiolucencies: 14, 16, 17, 26, 27, 36, 46

- Restorations:
  - 26 distal/occlusal/buccal/lingual: silver
  - 36 occlusal and buccal pit: silver
  - 46 occlusal: silver
- Calculus: Generalized moderate to heavy (distal 11, mesial 12, distal 25, mesial 31, mesial 32, mesial 41, distal 42, and mesial 46)

Q: What is your diagnosis of the patient?

Note: Always include a medical diagnosis when answering this question.

- Medical: American Society of Anesthesiologists (ASA) 1, healthy, past marijuana smoker (12 years)
- Periodontal: Generalized severe chronic periodontitis; American Academy of Periodontology (AAP) Type IV
- Dental
  - Parafunctional activity: Bruxism (sleeping)
  - Temporomandibular joint (TMJ)/musculature: No clicking or popping

Q: What etiology do you suspect to have caused this condition?

- Primary etiologic agent: Microbial plaque secondary to poor oral hygiene
- Distribution of plaque and calculus: Patient has generalized supra- and subgingival calculus
- Possible risk factors:
  - Genetics: No known occurrences of periodontal disease among family members
  - Poor oral hygiene
  - Smoking: Smoked marijuana two times per week for 12 years
  - Stress (coping)
  - Systemic factors: None

Q: What bacteria would you expect if you were to perform sensitivity testing?

Based on the diagnosis, one would expect *Prevotella intermedia, Tannerella forsythia,* and *Fusobacterium nucleatum.* The sensitivity testing confirmed this (Table 19-1). Clindamycin was prescribed based on the sensitivity testing.

Table 19-1 | Sensitivity testing results: Presumptive identification of periodontal pathogens*

Culture	Microbiota (%)	Inhibition (%)				
		Clindamycin	Amoxicillin	Metronidazole	Ciprofloxacin	Azithromycin
Aggregatibacter actinomycetemocomitans	0					
Porphyromonas gingivalis	0					
Prevotella intermedia	6.1	100	0	100	0	86
Tannerella forsythia	4.3	100	100	100	87	100
Campylobacter species	5.2	100	100	100	100	100
Eubacterium species	0					
Fusobacterium species	7.0	100	0	100	0	82
Peptostreptococcus micros	0					
Enteric gram-negative rods	0					
Beta hemolytic streptococci	0					
Yeast	0					
Eikenella corrodens	0					
Staphylococcus species	0					
Dialister pneumosintes	4.3	100	100	100	100	100

*Paper points placed on the mesial of 26 and 36.

Q: **What is the prognosis of the teeth in both the short and long term?**

- Overall: Fair (McGuire and Nunn classification[1])—The prognosis is highly dependent upon the strategic removal of the most compromised teeth, improved oral hygiene, and consistent preventive maintenance care.
- Individual short term (< 5 years):
  - Hopeless: 14
  - Poor: 11, 12, 16, 17, 21, 22, 31, 32, 38, 41, 42, 48
  - Fair: 26, 27, 36, 46
  - Good: 13, 23 to 25, 33, 37, 45, 47
- Individual long term (> 5 years):
  - Hopeless: 14, 38, 48
  - Poor: 11, 12, 16, 17, 21, 22, 31, 32, 41, 42
  - Fair: 24 to 27, 34 to 36, 44 to 46
  - Good: 13, 15, 23, 33, 37, 43, 47

Q: **What are your goals when strategizing the treatment plan for the patient?**

- Eradicate and change etiologic factors for periodontal disease
- Educate the patient on the causes and prevention of periodontal disease
- Improve oral hygiene and plaque control
- Reduce plaque and calculus to below disease threshold
- Establish and maintain the health of the periodontium
- Extract periodontally compromised teeth (14, 38, 48)
- Surgically reduce the deep periodontal pockets (more cleansable environment)
- Schedule regular periodontal maintenance recalls for monitoring and preventive care

Q: **What is your treatment plan for this patient?**

- Systemic: Encourage patient to maintain healthy lifestyle
- Diagnostic phase:
  - Emergency treatment: None
  - Examination
  - Diagnostic evaluation, study casts
  - Treatment plan/options presentation
  - Restorative consultation
- Preparatory phase:
  - Patient education/oral hygiene instructions (OHI)
  - Explanation of the disease etiology

- Current diagnosis and periodontal condition
- Explanation of risk factors: Poor oral hygiene
- Options: Nonsurgical vs surgical treatment vs extraction vs no treatment
- OHI: Modified Bass technique/interproximal brushes, rubber tip, and floss
• Phase I periodontal therapy (nonsurgical therapy):
- Microbiologic sensitivity testing
- Maxillary and mandibular left scaling and root planing (SRP)
- Maxillary and mandibular right SRP
- Periodontal reevaluation
• Surgical phase: Periodontal surgery:
- Extraction of 11 with socket preservation
- Pocket reduction for 23 to 27
- Pocket reduction for 34 to 37 and extraction of 38
- Pocket reduction for 15 to 17
- Pocket reduction for 43 to 47 and extraction of 48
• Maintenance phase:
- Supportive periodontal therapy with 3-month recall and monitoring

Results at reevaluation (Fig 19-4)

• Phase I therapy has been effective in this patient. Improvements in oral hygiene, reduction in pocket depths, and a decrease in marginal bleeding and increase in the percentage of teeth that are plaque free have all been observed.
• Oral hygiene improved, as noted by the increase in plaque-free areas (34% to 76%) and decrease in marginal bleeding index.
• A significant number of sites with pocket depth of 4 to 6 mm remained.

Fig 19-4 Reevaluation report record.

The chart shows an American Board of Periodontology Case Report Record.

AMERICAN BOARD OF PERIODONTOLOGY
CASE REPORT RECORD

Candidate Name: _____   Case Report No: _____

Patient's Number: _____   Age __36__ Sex _Male_ Race _Caucasion_

Stage of Therapy   Pre-Treatment   [Re-evaluation]   Post-treatment   Date of exam _____
(CIRCLE ONE)

Maxillary — Facial

	CAL & BOP	436	735	323		334	757	745	455	533	333		433	323	758	634	
	PD & Plaque	436	735	323		334	635	534	334	433	323		433	323	637	634	
	CEJ - GM	000	000	000		000	122	211	121	100	010		000	000	121	000	

Teeth: 2 3 4 | 6 7 8 9 10 11 | 12 13 14 15   FACIAL

Mobility Scale Used: __Miller__

Lingual mobility markings: +1 +1 +1 +1   LINGUAL

Maxillary — Lingual

	CEJ - GM		001	121	100		000	001	121	121	100	000		000	000	000	000	
	PD & Plaque		434	534	333		323	435	444	444	433	323		333	323	336	536	
	CAL & BOP		435	655	433		323	436	565	565	533	323		333	323	336	536	

Tooth numbers: 1 2 3 4 5 | 6 7 8 9 10 11 | 12 13 14 15 16

RIGHT _____ LEFT

Tooth numbers: 32 31 30 29 28 | 27 26 25 24 23 22 | 21 20 19 18 17

Mandibular — Facial

	CAL & BOP	344	565	734	333	325	446	565	544	644	438	333	433	326	436	435	533
	PD & Plaque	444	444	734	333	324	334	333	433	533	327	333	433	326	436	435	534
	CEJ - GM	-100	121	000	000	001	112	232	111	111	111	000	000	000	000	000	00-1

Teeth: 32 31 30 29 28 | 27 26 25 24 23 22 | 21 20 19   FACIAL

Furcation Grade System Used: **Glickmann**

Lingual mobility markings: +1 +1 +1 +1   LINGUAL

Mandibular — Lingual

	CEJ - GM	-100	000	000	000	000	000	000	000	000	000	000	000	000	000	000	00-1
	PD & Plaque	765	446	636	634	533	323	433	323	333	335	544	434	336	447	445	645
	CAL & BOP	665	446	636	634	533	323	433	323	333	335	544	434	336	447	445	644

Q: What is your rationale for surgical pocket reduction therapy?

- Surgical pocket reduction therapy was indicated because of the high number of remaining deep periodontal pockets and for further removal of calculus and its associated subgingival microflora. This may provide improvements in clinical attachment level, minimize further inflammation, and achieve reduction and stability in probing depths for supportive periodontal therapy.
- Goals of surgical therapy:
  - Provide access to the roots for effective plaque and calculus removal
  - Decrease remaining pocket depths through soft tissue reduction and osseous recontouring
  - Allow for oral hygiene access for the patient and periodontist
- Stambaugh et al[2] showed that trained hygienists who scaled teeth under local anesthesia achieved a "curet efficiency" of 3.73 mm. The instrument limit where evidence of instrumentation could be seen was 6.21 mm.
- Caffesse et al[3] noted that while scaling only and scaling with a flap increased the percentage of root surface without calculus, scaling following the reflection of a flap aided calculus removal in pockets 4 mm and deeper. Percentages of tooth surfaces completely free of calculus following scaling only versus scaling with a flap, respectively, at various pocket depths were 86% versus 86% for 1- to 3-mm pockets, 43% versus 76% for 4- to 6-mm pockets, and 32% versus 50% for > 6–mm pockets.

Q: Please show and describe how you would extract tooth 14 and graft the site.

Figure 19-5 shows the radiographic appearance of tooth 14 before extraction. The surgical procedure was performed as follows:

- Buccal: A sulcular incision was made from the facial of tooth 16 to the mesial aspect of tooth 13 (Fig 19-6a).
- Palatal: A sulcular incision was made from the palatal of tooth 16 to the mesial aspect of tooth 13 (Fig 19-6b).
- The tooth was extracted. No buccal plate was evident (Fig 19-6c).
- Soft tissue and granulation removal were performed, followed by thorough SRP with hand instruments. Freeze-dried bone allograft (FDBA) was placed into the defect with two layers of Bio-Gide membrane (Geistlich) because of the lack of a buccal plate (Fig 19-6d).
- Interrupted sutures (Gore-Tex, W. L. Gore) were placed from the mesial aspect of tooth 15 to the distal aspect of tooth 13 (Figs 19-6e and 19-6f).
- The patient was given one tablet of ibuprofen (800 mg) and an ice pack. He was also prescribed 500 mg amoxicillin three times per day for 1 week.

Fig 19-5 Radiograph of tooth 14 showing gutta-percha extending to the apex.

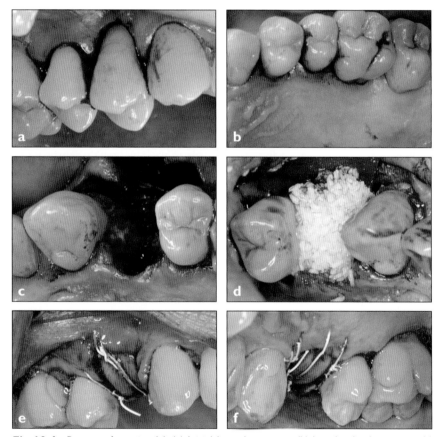

Fig 19-6 Bone graft at site 14. (*a*) Initial buccal incisions. (*b*) Initial palatal incisions. (*c*) Extraction of the tooth. (*d*) Placement of bone graft and membrane. (*e*) Buccal view of sutures. (*f*) Lingual view of sutures.

Q: Provide the rationale for the choice of graft and barrier.

Graft
- Mellonig[4] demonstrated complete or greater than 50% bone fill in 67% of sites treated with FDBA alone and in 78% of sites treated with FDBA and autogenous bone.
- A 2005 AAP position paper[5] found bone fill ranging from 1.3 to 2.6 mm when FDBA was used to treat defects. Human trials using demineralized FDBA (DFDBA) have demonstrated bone fill similar to that achieved with FDBA, ranging from 1.7 to 2.9 mm.
- Comparisons between bone allografts and alloplasts suggest that they produce similar clinical results.[5]
- A meta-analysis by Vignoletti et al[6] found that socket preservation therapies resulted in significantly less vertical and horizontal contraction of the alveolar bone crest.

Barrier
- The membrane will prevent apical migration of the epithelium and protect the wound.
- Resorbable membrane: Laurell et al[7] reviewed studies presented during the last 20 years on the surgical treatment of intrabony defects, analyzing treatment results of open-flap debridement, bone replacement grafts, and guided tissue regeneration. No difference was found between resorbable and nonresorbable membranes.

Q: Discuss implant placement in site 14.

- Study casts and photographs are important for planning treatment when the patient is not present.
- Cone beam computed tomography (CBCT) scans are necessary to determine the height of available bone in three dimensions and therefore to select the appropriate implant. They also may be needed to determine the location of anatomical structures (ie, nerves, vessels, and the sinus).
- Written informed consent is discussed between the surgeon and the patient.
- Figure 19-7 presents the implant placement procedures.

After the patient has been anesthetized, a full-thickness incision is made in KAT in the edentulous area. A vertical incision may be needed for reflection.

A periosteal elevator is used to raise the flap. Great care must be taken to avoid any tears in the flap.

After the bone is exposed, the implants are placed based on manufacturer recommendation (direction indicators and radiographs should be taken to ensure proper angulation).

A cover screw or healing abutment is placed and the flaps are sutured.

Fig 19-7 Implant placement procedures. KAT—keratinized attached tissue.

Q: Describe your technique for performing osseous resective surgery on the maxillary left quadrant.

The procedures for resective osseous surgery in the maxillary left quadrant are presented in Fig 19-8 and outlined below:

1. Buccal: A sulcular incision is made from the facial of tooth 23 to the distofacial aspect of tooth 27 (see Fig 19-8c).
2. Palatal: A sulcular incision is made from the mesial aspect of tooth 23 to the distal aspect of tooth 27 (see Fig 19-8d). (A distal wedge incision is made on the distal aspect of tooth 27.)
3. Full-thickness reflection is performed, followed by degranulation and SRP using Cavitron (Dentsply) and hand instruments (see Figs 19-8e and 19-8f).
4. Osteoplasty and ostectomy are done with a handpiece and hand instruments to maintain positive architecture (see Figs 19-8g and 19-8h).
5. The buccal and lingual flaps are sutured with interrupted (chromic gut) sutures (see Figs 19-8i and 19-8j).
6. Coe-Pak (GC) is placed, and the patient is prescribed ibuprofen 800 mg (1 tablet every 6 hours) as an anti-inflammatory and for pain management. Adequate postoperative healing is noted at the follow-up appointment.

Fig 19-8 *(a)* Initial buccal view. *(b)* Initial palatal view. *(c)* Initial buccal incisions. *(d)* Initial palatal incisions. *(e)* Buccal view before osseous resective surgery. *(f)* Palatal view before osseous resective surgery. *(g)* Buccal view following osseous resective surgery. *(h)* Palatal view following osseous resective surgery. *(i)* Buccal sutures. *(j)* Palatal sutures.

Q: **Discuss the reasoning behind using a dressing, and then explain why a surgeon may decide not to use a dressing.**

Figure 19-9 presents the rationale for placing or not placing a dressing.

Placing
- Protects the wound
- Increases patient comfort
- Stabilizes the flap
- Retains the graft material

Not placing
- Increases postoperative pain
- Irritates
- Increases plaque retention (increased bacteria): Powell et al[8] found that the use of a postsurgical dressing demonstrated a slightly higher rate of infection (8 infections in 300 procedures, 2.67%) than nonuse of a dressing (14 infections in 753 procedures, 1.86%)

Fig 19-9 Rationale for placing or not placing a dressing.

Q: **Describe the specific technique for the treatment of teeth 43 to 48.**

Procedures for resective osseous surgery in the mandibular right quadrant and extraction of tooth 48 are presented in Fig 19-10 and described below:

1. Buccal: A sulcular incision is made from the facial of tooth 43 to the distal aspect of tooth 48 (see Fig 19-10c).
2. Lingual: A sulcular incision is made from the lingual of tooth 43 to the mesial aspect of tooth 48 (see Fig 19-10d).
3. Full-thickness reflection is performed, followed by degranulation and SRP using Cavitron and hand instruments (see Figs 19-10e and 19-10f).
4. Tooth 48 is extracted, and ostectomy is performed with a handpiece and hand instruments between teeth 46 and 47 and between teeth 45 and 46 (see Figs 19-10g and 19-10h).
5. The buccal and lingual flaps are sutured with interrupted (silk) sutures (see Figs 19-10i and 19-10j).
6. Coe-Pak is placed, and the patient is prescribed ibuprofen 800 mg (1 tablet every 6 hours) as an anti-inflammatory and for pain management. Adequate postoperative healing is noted at the follow-up appointment.

Fig 19-10 *(a)* Initial buccal view. *(b)* Initial lingual view. *(c)* Initial buccal incisions. *(d)* Initial lingual incisions. *(e)* Buccal view before osseous resective surgery. *(f)* Lingual view before osseous resective surgery. *(g)* Buccal sutures. *(h)* Lingual sutures.

Q: What instructions should be provided to the patient after surgery?

Figure 19-11 presents instructions that should be provided to the patient after surgery.

Care of your mouth: Immediately after surgery, keep ice cold water or other cold foods such as ice cream or frozen yogurt in your mouth for 6 to 8 hours. Do not brush your teeth in the areas that have dressing or sutures. Do all normal cleaning of teeth that did not undergo surgery.

Activity: Reduce your activity following surgery. No running, weight lifting, or any strenuous aerobic activity or contact sports for 48 hours.

Discomfort: Following all types of surgery, you can expect some discomfort. Take pain medication as prescribed; do not drink alcoholic beverages in combination with pain medication.

Swelling: In some cases swelling may be expected, but it will go away in 3 to 4 days.

Eating: Eat only cold, soft foods on the day of surgery. After the first day, stay on a soft but balanced diet. Do not eat hard, crunchy, or spicy foods.

Smoking: Do not smoke following surgery. Tobacco smoke is an irritant and delays healing of the tissue. Refrain from smoking for as long as possible.

Fig 19-11 Postoperative instructions.

Q: What factors would you consider when evaluating the results of therapy?

1. Examination
• Periodontal tissues
  - Color: Pink fibrotic tissue
  - Texture: Generalized firm tissue
  - Tone: Gingival tissues are generally fibrotic
• Probing depths: Generalized 2- to 5-mm pockets with localized 6-mm pockets (Table 19-2 and Fig 19-12)

Table 19-2 Results of therapy

Parameter	Initial	Reevalutaion	Postsurgery
Marginal bleeding	14%	6%	5%
Plaque-free areas	34%	76%	87%
Pockets > 3 mm with BOP	17%	12%	11%
Pockets < 3 mm	78 (43%)	92 (54%)	126 (78%)
Pockets 4 to 6 mm	91 (51%)	74 (43%)	34 (21%)
Pockets > 6 mm	10 (6%)	6 (3%)	2 (1%)

AMERICAN BOARD OF PERIODONTOLOGY
CASE REPORT RECORD

Candidate Name: _____ Case Report No: _____
Patient's Number: _____ Age _36_ Sex _Male_ Race _Caucasion_

Stage of Therapy   Pre-Treatment   Re-evaluation   [Post-treatment]   Date of exam _____
(CIRCLE ONE)

CAL & BOP	445	848	323			324	456	744	445	533	343		323	323	457	635	
PD & Plaque	445	544	323			324	334	433	324	433	333		323	323	336	635	
CEJ - GM	000	303	000			000	122	311	121	100	010		000	000	121	000	

FACIAL

Mobility Scale
Used: __Miller__

LINGUAL

CEJ - GM		001	121	100			000	001	121	121	100	000		000	000	020	010	
PD & Plaque		335	534	323			323	323	443	333	323	323		333	323	334	544	
CAL & BOP		336	655	423			323	324	564	454	423	323		333	323	354	554	
	1	2	3	4	5	6	7	8	9	10	11	12	13	14	15	16

RIGHT _____ LEFT

	32	31	30	29	28	27	26	25	24	23	22	21	20	19	18	17
CAL & BOP		455	633	323	344		555	565	545	545	547	556		334	323	456	546	
PD & Plaque		334	433	323	323		323	333	323	323	325	334		334	323	334	335	
CEJ - GM		121	200	000	021		232	232	222	222	222	222		000	000	122	211	

FACIAL

Furcation Grade
System Used:
Glickmann

LINGUAL

CEJ - GM		121	221	000	000		000	000	121	121	121	010		000	000	000	000	
PD & Plaque		334	633	323	323		222	222	222	222	224	323		333	334	435	444	
CAL & BOP		455	854	323	323		222	222	343	343	345	333		333	334	435	444	

Fig 19-12 Posttreatment report record.

- Recession: Generalized moderate recession on 11, 12, 21 to 23, 26, 31, 32, 41 to 44, and 47 (Fig 19-13)
- Mobility: Miller Class I: 11, 12, 21, 22, 31, 32, 41, and 42

Fig 19-13 Intraoral frontal view following periodontal therapy.

Fig 19-14 Posttreatment radiographs.

- Furcation (Glickman):
  - Grade I: 27B, 37B, and 47B
  - Grade II: 16B, 16ML, 16DL, 17B, 17DL, 26B, 26DL, 36BL, and 46B
  - Grade III: None

2. Sensitivity testing

The antibiotic regimen (clindamycin) in conjunction with the periodontal therapy was successful in reducing the periodontal pathogens in the mouth. No more microbiota were found in the final sensitivity testing.

3. Radiographs

Although the radiographs show bone loss, it has improved, and no calculus is shown (Fig 19-14).

Fig 19-15 *(a to h)* Intraoral views following treatment.

4. Photographs
The photographs show pink, healthy tissues with no plaque or calculus present (Fig 19-15).

5. All three goals of surgical therapy (see question on page 255) have been met:
- Provide access to the roots for effective plaque and calculus removal
- Decrease remaining pocket depths through soft tissue reduction and osseous recontouring
- Allow for oral hygiene access for the patient and periodontist

Q: What factors would you consider in developing an optimal maintenance schedule for this patient?

Following are the factors to be considered in developing an optimal maintenance schedule[9]:

- BOP greater than 25% (patient has 11%)
- Pocket depth (patient has localized areas with greater than 4-mm probing depth)
- Tooth loss (patient is missing four teeth)
- Age in relation to loss of periodontal support (patient is young)
- Systemic and genetic factors (none reported)
- Environment (history of smoking)
- Oral hygiene (poor)
- Compliance (patient is much more compliant)

Studies have reported that patients who have had a history of periodontal disease need to be recalled at least four times per year.[10]

Q: If the mandibular right quadrant started to show further bone loss in 10 years, would you re-treat it?

Note: There is no wrong answer, but the answer will need to be supported by logical thinking.

Yes, there was a study done that found that nearly half of the patients who were originally treated for periodontal disease and consistently kept their follow-up appointments needed retreatment at least once during a 13-year period. Comprehensive maintenance care and surgical retreatments appeared to limit additional tooth loss for patients at risk because of indeterminate or poor preliminary prognosis, erratic or poor compliance, and a family history of periodontal disease.[11]

Case 2

Patient identification

- Age: 43 years
- Sex: Male
- Ethnicity: Indian
- No history of smoking

History of present illness

Chief complaint: Maxillary anterior teeth "are getting more loose every day" (Fig 19-16).

Fig 19-16 Frontal view with the jaws closed *(a)* and with the jaws open *(b)*.

Medical history

- General health: Good
- Medications: None
- Allergies: None

Family history
- Diabetes: None
- Cardiovascular disease: None
- Bleeding disorders: None
- Tuberculosis: None
- Mental/emotional disorders: None
- Periodontal disease: None

Dental history

- Restorative experience: Minimal (see Fig 19-16b)
- Orthodontics: None reported
- Frequency of prior care: Infrequent
- Oral hygiene: Fair
  - Brushing: Twice a day
  - Flossing: Twice a day

Clinical examination

Dental examination
- Missing: 18, 28, and 38
- Wear facets/attrition: Generalized moderate occlusal and incisal wear
- Abrasion: None
- Abfraction: None
- Parafunctional activity: Suspected clenching/grinding
- Staining: Moderate generalized staining
- Display at rest: Maxillary teeth 1 to 2 mm (Fig 19-17a)
- Display during smiling: Maxillary teeth to first molar, 1 to 2 mm of gingival tissue and mandibular teeth (Fig 19-17b)

Fig 19-17 Patient at rest *(a)* and smiling *(b)*.

Fig 19-18 Posterior occlusion.

Occlusal examination
- Angle classification: Dental molar Class I (Fig 19-18)
- Canine relationship: Class I on both sides
- Centric relation: Repeatable
- Left lateral guidance: Group
- Right lateral guidance: Group
- Incisal relationship:
  - Horizontal overlap: 5 to 6 mm (because of the mobility of tooth 11)
  - Vertical overlap: 3 mm (tooth 11 supererupted)

Periodontal examination
- Plaque/calculus: Generalized heavy plaque with heavy supragingival and sub-gingival calculus
- Oral hygiene: Poor
- Plaque free: 65% (initial)
- Marginal bleeding: 25% (initial)
- Periodontal tissues: Generalized areas of compromised tissue with local-ized moderate to severe cyanotic areas and blunted papilla
- Probing depths: Generalized 3 to 9 mm
- BOP: Localized
- Recession (Miller):
  - Class 2: 13, 23
  - Class 3: 11, 12, 21, 22
- Mobility (Miller):
  - Class II: 12, 22
  - Class III: 11, 21

Fig 19-19 Pretreatment radiographs.

Radiographic examination
- Bone loss: Generalized moderate horizontal bone loss with localized vertical defects (Fig 19-19)
- Radiolucencies: 11
- Calculus: Generalized moderate to heavy deposits

Q: What is your diagnosis of the patient?

- Medical: ASA 1, healthy
- Periodontal: Generalized moderate chronic periodontitis and localized severe chronic periodontitis with BOP (patient may have had aggressive periodontitis when he was younger); AAP Type III
- Mucogingival deformities and conditions around teeth: Gingival/soft tissue recession on the facial or lingual surfaces of the maxillary anterior teeth

Fig 19-20 Intraoral lateral view of teeth in occlusion.

Q: What is the etiology of the bone loss?

- Primary etiologic agent: Microbial plaque secondary to poor oral hygiene
- Distribution of plaque and calculus: Generalized supra- and subgingival calculus (Fig 19-20)
- Possible risk factors:
  - Genetics: No known occurrences of periodontal disease among family members
  - Poor oral hygiene
  - Stress (coping)
  - Systemic factors: None

Q: What is the prognosis for the maxillary incisors?

Based on the classification by Kwok and Caton,[12] the prognosis is unfavorable. There are many local factors that indicate an unfavorable prognosis for these teeth:

- Deep probing depths and attachment loss
- Anatomical plaque-related factors (open contacts)
- Class II and Class III mobility

Q: What are the treatment options for the maxillary incisors?

Figure 19-21 presents the treatment options for the maxillary incisors.

Option 1: No further treatment

Option 2: Implants
1. Preoperative assessment/diagnostic information
   • Wax-up
   • Fabrication of surgical stent
   • CT scan
2. Bone graft/soft tissue augmentation
3. Implant-supported fixed partial denture (11, 12, 21, 22)

Option 3: Fixed partial denture (canine to canine)

Option 4: Maxillary removable partial denture

Fig 19-21 Treatment options for the maxillary incisors.

Q: You indicated that a bone graft would most likely be needed before implant placement. What are the options for a horizontal bone graft?

- Socket grafting: Placing a bone graft into the socket may allow for preservation of the ridge in the esthetic zone
- Bone and membrane guided bone regeneration using FDBA or DFDBA
- Autogenous block graft (eg, tuberosity, chin, and lateral ramus)
- Ridge splitting: May reduce treatment time and morbidity
- Distraction osteogenesis: No graft requirement and concurrent enlargement of soft tissue
- Block allograft: Not living bone, must be hydrated, and air bubbles must be removed

Q: Which option did you choose and why?

Note: There is no wrong answer to this question as long as it is well supported.

FDBA and a resorbable membrane were used to horizontally augment the ridge in preparation for implants. The CBCT scan shows that the buccal plate is not thick enough in the esthetic area to allow proper implant placement (Fig 19-22). According to Beitlitum et al,[13] good clinical results can be achieved by placing FDBA and barrier membranes to treat large vertical and/or horizontal ridge deficiencies. Geurs et al[14] found that lateral alveolar ridge augmentation resulting from the use of a synthetic long-term resorbable membrane and an allograft was comparable to that obtained using other materials while avoiding the need to harvest a graft or perform a second surgery to remove the membrane.

Fig 19-22 *(a)* Extraction of the maxillary incisors. *(b)* Clinical view of the ridge before bone graft placement, 7 months after extraction. *(c)* CBCT scans of implant position for site 12. *(d)* CBCT scans of implant position for site 22.

Q: **Describe your technique for grafting the anterior maxilla.**

Incisions were made in keratinized tissue, and a flap was reflected. The Bio-Gide membrane was cut to fit the site, and FDBA was placed under the membrane. The anterior maxilla was then sutured with silk and Gore-Tex sutures using the horizontal matress and interrupted suture technique (Fig 19-23).

Fig 19-23 Bone graft surgery. *(a)* Initial incisions for bone graft placement. *(b)* FDBA placement. *(c)* Membrane positioning. *(d)* Suture placement. *(e)* One month postoperative. *(f)* Initial incisions for implant placement. *(g)* Bone morphology before implant placement. *(h)* Direction indicators placed before implant placement. *(i)* Implants placed. *(j)* Sutures (Gore-Tex) positioned. *(k)* Three months after implant placement. *(l)* One year after implant placement.

Q: **What should be evaluated when placing the anterior implants?**

The following should be included in the evaluation prior to placing anterior implants[15]:

- Mesiodistal dimension of the edentulous area
- Three-dimensional (3D) imaging of the site
- Neighboring teeth (tooth dimensions, form, position, and orientation; periodontal/endodontic status; length of roots; crown-to-root ratio)
- Interarch relationships (vertical dimension of occlusion, interocclusal space)
- Esthetic parameters (height of upper smile line, lower lip line, occlusal plane orientation, dental and facial symmetry)
- Patient expectations
- Oral hygiene
- Primary stability of the implants

Q: **Discuss implant placement in the esthetic area.**

- Low trauma
- Precise 3D positioning
- Slightly palatal positioning to preserve keratinized tissue on the labial aspect
- Use of a screw-retained implant to prevent subgingival cement placement
- Deeper placement of the implants in sites 12 and 22 to allow the superstructure to be hidden and a gradual emergence profile

Q: **How will you evaluate the success of the implants at maintenance visits?**[16,17]

The following parameters are used to evaluate the success of implants[16,17]:

- The implants should be immobile (less than 1 mm in any direction) and functioning
- Radiographs show no radiolucency
  - Vertical bone loss is less than 0.2 mm annually following the implant's first year of service
  - Implant has no persistent and/or irreversible signs
  - Patient and clinician are satisfied
  - The hard and soft tissues are healthy

Fig 19-24 Abscess on the buccal aspect of the mandibular right second molar.

Case 3

The patient is a 65-year-old white man complaining of oral malodor. His dentist referred him to you to access the mandibular right second molar because of swelling, pus, and soreness. When he sits in your chair, he seems disoriented and irritable. When you look in his mouth, you find generalized inflammation of the gingiva and an abscess on the buccal aspect of the mandibular right second molar with suppuration (Fig 19-24). Charting demonstrates an 8-mm facial pocket and 6-mm palatal and interproximal pockets.

Q: What is your diagnosis of the patient?

Medical
There are a number of reasons for the patient to appear dazed and irritable:

- Hypoglycemia or hyperglycemia
- Alcohol or drug overdose
- Hyperthyroidism or hypothyroidism
- Cerebrovascular incident

Dental
- The patient may have diabetes mellitus–associated gingivitis related to the endocrine system, under the heading of gingival diseases modified by systemic diseases, which is a subcategory of dental plaque–induced gingival diseases.
- The patient has a periodontal abscess, which is a subclassification of abscesses of the periodontium.

Q: What could have led to the abscess formation?

- Diabetes: According to Bjelland et al,[18] multiple periodontal abscesses may result from uncontrolled hyperglycemia. Rees[19] listed multiple or recurrent periodontal abscesses among the possible indications of undiagnosed or poorly controlled diabetes mellitus.

- The abscess may also be caused by a preexisting periodontal pocket in association with bacteria at the depth of the pocket.
- A foreign body can also cause a periodontal abscess.

Q: How will you treat the periodontal abscess?

- I would ask the patient if he has seen his physician recently and whether he knows his hemoglobin A_{1c} levels to determine if the abscess may be associated with diabetes (only his medical doctor can make that diagnosis).
- An incision at a 90-degree angle to the long axis of the tooth will drain the exudate. Without removal of the cause (foreign body, bacteria, or calculus), the abscess will recur. If this is not possible, extraction might be necessary.[20]
- Antibiotics and analgesics should be prescribed. A follow-up with a dentist is also needed.[21]

Fig 19-25 Clinical view of the patient's palate.

Case 4

An 80-year-old patient presents to the office with a chief complaint of a continuous burning feeling on his palate (Fig 19-25). Upon examination you find that the patient is extremely sensitive. When you finish your examination, the patient complains of sudden chest pain. He starts to sweat and has labored breathing.

Q: What is your diagnosis of the patient?

- Medical: There are a number of possibilities for the patient to have chest pain and labored breathing. The patient might be experiencing an acute myocardial infarction, hyperventilation, or angina pectoris.

- Dental: The patient has a *Candida* species infection, which is a gingival disease of fungal origin. It is also known as *atrophic (erythematous) candidiasis*.

Q: How will you manage the patient if he is having a myocardial infarction?

1. Stop the dental procedure
2. Administer oxygen to the patient at 4 to 6 liters per minute
3. Call 911
4. Administer nitroglycerin from the emergency kit (if pain continues, most likely not angina)
5. Administer aspirin (fibrinolytic properties)
6. Monitor vital signs
7. Manage the patient's pain with opioids (morphine) or nitrous oxide

Q: What is your approach to treating the dental condition of this patient?

I would first treat the condition with a topical antifungal (eg, nystatin or clotrimazole troches) applied to the tissue side of the denture four to six times a day for 2 to 3 weeks. If the fungal infection persists, I would treat the patient with 100 mg fluconazole daily.

References

1. McGuire MK. Prognosis versus actual outcome: A long-term survey of 100 treated periodontal patients under maintenance care. J Periodontol 1991;62:51–58.
2. Stambaugh RV, Dragoo M, Smith DM, Carasali L. The limits of subgingival scaling. Int J Periodontics Restorative Dent 1981;1(5):30–41.
3. Caffesse RG, Sweeney PL, Smith BA. Scaling and root planing with and without periodontal flap surgery. J Clin Periodontol 1986;13:205–210.
4. Mellonig JT. Freeze-dried bone allografts in periodontal reconstructive surgery. Dent Clin North Am 1991;35:505–520.
5. Wang HL, Greenwell H, Fiorellini W; Research, Schience and Therapy Committee of the American Academy of Periodontolgy. Position paper: Periodontal regeneration. J Periodontol 2005;76:1601–1622.
6. Vignoletti F, Matesanz P, Rodrigo D, Figuero E, Martin C, Sanz M. Surgical protocols for ridge preservation after tooth extraction. A systematic review. Clin Oral Implants Res 2012;23(suppl 5):22–38.
7. Laurell L, Gottlow J, Zybutz M, Persson R. Treatment of intrabony defects by different surgical procedures. A literature review. J Periodontol 1998;69:303–313.
8. Powell CA, Mealey BL, Deas DE, McDonnell HT, Moritz AJ. Post-surgical infections: Prevalence associated with various periodontal surgical procedures. J Periodontol 2005;76:329–333.
9. Lang NP, Brägger U, Salvi GE, Tonetti MS. Supportive periodontal therapy (SPT). In: Lindhe J, Lang NP, Karring T. Clinical Periodontology and Implant Dentistry, ed 5. Oxford, UK: Blackwell Munksgaard 2008:1303.
10. Cohen RE; Research, Science and Therapy Committee of the American Academy of Periodontology. Position paper: Periodontal maintenance. J Periodontol 2003;74:1395–1401.

11. Fardal O, Linden GJ. Re-treatment profiles during long-term maintenance therapy in a periodon-tal practice in Norway. J Clin Periodontol 2005;32:744–749.

12. Kwok V, Caton JG. Commentary: Prognosis revisited: A system for assigning periodontal progno-sis. J Periodontol 2007;78:2063–2071.

13. Beitlitum I, Artzi Z, Nemcovsky CE. Clinical evaluation of particulate allogeneic with and without autogenous bone grafts and resorbable collagen membranes for bone augmentation of atrophic alveolar ridges. Clin Oral Implants Res 2010;21:1242–1250.

14. Geurs NC, Korostoff JM, Vassilopoulos PJ, et al. Clinical and histologic assessment of lateral al-veolar ridge augmentation using a synthetic long-term bioabsorbable membrane and an allograft. J Periodontol 2008;79:1133–1140.

15. Cortellini P, Tonetti MS. Regenerative periodontal therapy. In: Lindhe J, Lang NP, Karring T. Clini-cal Periodontology and Implant Dentistry, ed 5. Oxford, UK: Blackwell Munksgaard 2008:918.

16. Zarb GA, Albrektsson T. Criteria for determining clinical success with osseointegrated dental implants [in French]. Cah Prothese 1990;(71):19–26.

17. Cochran DL. A comparison of endosseous dental implant surfaces. J Periodontol 1999;70:1523–1539.

18. Bjelland S, Bray P, Gupta N, Hirscht R. Dentists, diabetes and periodontitis. Aust Dent J 2002;47:202–207.

19. Rees TD. Periodontal management of the patient with diabetes mellitus. Periodontol 2000 2000;23:63–72.

20. Sivapathasundharam B. Diseases of the periodontium. In: Rajendran R, Sivapathasundharam B (eds). Shafer's Textbook of Oral Pathology, ed 6. New Delhi: Elsevier, 2009:404.

21. DeFlitch CJ. Throat and oropharynx. In: Aghababian R (ed). Essentials of Emergency Medicine. Sudbury, MA: Jones and Bartlett, 2006:238.

Index